BODY SIGNS

How to Be

Your Own

Diagnostic

Detective

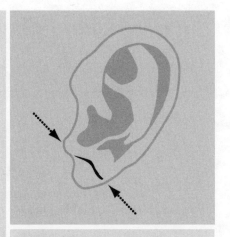

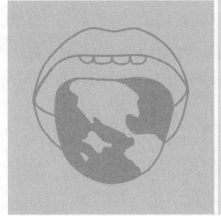

BODY SIGNS

Joan Liebmann-Smith, Ph. D.,
and Jacqueline Nardi Egan

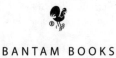

BANTAM BOOKS

New York Toronto London Sydney Auckland

BODY SIGNS: HOW TO BE YOUR OWN DIAGNOSTIC DETECTIVE
A Bantam Book / January 2008

Published by Bantam Dell
A Division of Random House, Inc.
New York, New York

Book design by Ellen Cipriano

Cover and interior illustrations copyright © 2007 by Nenad Jakesevic

Library of Congress Cataloging-in-Publication Data

Liebmann-Smith, Joan.
    Body signs : how to be your own diagnostic detective / Joan Liebmann-Smith and Jacqueline Nardi Egan.
        p. cm.
    ISBN 978-0-553-80507-9 (hardcover)
    1. Symptoms—Popular works. 2. Medicine, Popular. I. Egan, Jacqueline Nardi. II. Title.

RC69.L54 2008
616'.047—dc22   2007028576

Printed in the United States of America
Published simultaneously in Canada

www.bantamdell.com

10 9 8 7 6 5 4 3 2 1
BVG

To the memory of my parents, John and Dorothy Liebmann, both of whom died prematurely of heart disease because they and their doctors missed the warning and danger signs.

And to Richard and Rebecca, who keep my heart beating with happiness.

Joan Liebmann-Smith

To the memory of my husband, Edward, a sign that eternal love is possible; and to our daughter, Elizabeth, who continues to be a sign that hope and joy exist.

Jacqueline Nardi Egan

ACKNOWLEDGMENTS

First and foremost, we want to thank our incomparable agent Kris Dahl for loving the idea of *Body Signs* as much as we did, and Jim Gorman for putting us in touch with Kris. And we're very grateful to Bantam Books for embracing *Body Signs* with such enthusiasm. We couldn't have asked for a better editor than Beth Rashbaum. Beth's outstanding editing skills, her kind, gentle prodding, and her sense of humor made working with her a pleasure. She; her assistant, Meghan Keenan; the production editor, Kelly Chian; and the art director, Paolo Pepe, were wonderfully helpful, supportive, and understanding in dealing with all our eccentricities and occasional testiness. *Body Signs* will be read around the world thanks to the tireless efforts of Sharon Swados and Lisa George in the subsidiary-rights division, who realized its universal appeal and spread the word.

We're indebted to Nenad Jakesevic for his terrific book jacket and chapter illustrations, and to his fellow artist and wife, Sonja Lamut, for her aesthetic input. And thanks to Michael Raab for the flattering photo.

We're very grateful to the members of our distinguished panel of medical experts for their help, comments, and input: Dr. Pete S. Batra, Dr.

Wilma Bergfeld, Dr. Michael Bloom, Dr. Stephen DiMartino, Dr. Loren W. Greene, Dr. Axel Grothey, Dr. Stuart I. Henochowicz, Dr. Gordon Hughes, Dr. Alan Kominsky, Dr. Ronald Kraft, Dr. Sharon Lewin, Dr. Larry Lipshultz, Dr. Michael Osborne, Dr. Shelley Peck, Dr. Rock Positano, Dr. Joseph Scharpf, Dr. John Stangel, Dr. Randall Zusman, and Dr. Michael Bloom.

Many thanks to Richard Liebmann-Smith for his superb editorial input, not to mention his soups, stews, and sauces. And thanks to Rebecca Liebmann-Smith for her suggestions and editing skills, which someday soon may surpass even her father's; and to Elizabeth Egan Serraillier, M.P.H., who never let us forget how important it is to educate people about their health.

Mary Diamond, Barbara Kantrowitz, Dr. Kenneth Magid, Susan Orlins, Eliza Orlins, Steve Price, and Dr. Laura Sternberg provided us with help in a variety of ways. And a special thanks to Jonathan Schwartz, whose National Public Radio show made working on weekend afternoons tolerable, if not enjoyable.

Finally, a big thank-you to our friends and relatives, who bombarded us with their bizarre body signs and—more important—their love, support, and understanding when we had to decline or cancel social engagements.

CONTENTS

CHAPTER 3. LISTENING TO YOUR EARS 67

Red Ears ▪ Earlobe Crease ▪ Misshapen Ears ▪ Too Much Earwax ▪ Watery Ear Discharge ▪ Itchy Ears ▪ Stuffy Ears ▪ Ringing in Your Ears ▪ Hearing Your Heartbeat ▪ Sensitivity to Sound ▪ Hearing a Loud Explosion When Sleeping ▪ Hearing Sounds That Others Don't ▪ Gradual Hearing Loss ▪ Sudden Hearing Loss

CHAPTER 4. YOUR NOSE KNOWS 83

A Red Nose ▪ A Bulbous Nose ▪ A Crease over the Nose ▪ Sun Sneezing ▪ Inability to Sneeze ▪ Snoring ▪ A Very Runny Nose ▪ A Dry Nose ▪ A Smelly Nose ▪ Smelling Problems

CHAPTER 5. READ MY LIPS . . . AND MOUTH 99

Puffy Lips ▪ Pursed Lips ▪ Dry, Cracked Lips ▪ Blue Lips ▪ Burning, Tingling Lips or Mouth ▪ Lip or Mouth Freckles ▪ White or Gray Patches in Your Mouth ▪ White Streaks in the Mouth ▪ Red or Swollen Gums ▪ A Bump or Hole on the Roof of Your Mouth ▪ A Dry Mouth or Excessive Thirst ▪ Watery Mouth ▪ Black Hairy Tongue ▪ White Hairy Tongue ▪ Beefy Red Tongue ▪ Groovy Tongue ▪ A Smooth Tongue ▪ Traveling Tongue Patches ▪ Twitchy Tongue ▪ Diminished or Distorted Sense of Taste ▪ A Metallic or Terrible Taste ▪ Supersensitive Taste ▪ Sweet, Fruity Breath ▪ Garlic Breath ▪ Urine- or Ammonia-Smelling Breath ▪ Fishy Breath ▪ Fecal Breath ▪ Yellow-Brown Teeth ▪ Greenish or Metallic-Colored Teeth ▪ Bluish Gray Teeth ▪ Spotted Teeth ▪ Blackish Teeth ▪ Indented or Notched Teeth ▪ Smooth, Glassy-Looking Teeth ▪ Cracked Teeth

CHAPTER 6. TELLING THE TRUTH: YOUR THROAT, VOICE, NECK, AND JAW 129

Lumps on the Front of the Neck ▪ Lumps Elsewhere on the Neck ▪ A Lump in the Throat ▪ A Lump on the Jaw ▪ Clicking Jaw ▪ Stiff Jaw ▪ Receding or Thrusting Chin ▪ Frequent Yawning ▪ Excessive Hiccupping ▪ Chronic

Coughing ▪ Colored Phlegm ▪ A Hoarse, Raspy Voice ▪ A Sporadically Hoarse Voice ▪ Frequent Throat Clearing ▪ Trembly Voice ▪ Slurred Speech ▪ Suddenly Speaking with a Foreign Accent ▪ Speaking Too Loudly or Too Softly

CHAPTER 7. THE MAIN BODY OF EVIDENCE: YOUR TORSO AND EXTREMITIES   151

Mismatched Breasts ▪ A Lump in the Breast ▪ Lumpy Breasts ▪ Swollen, Discolored Breasts ▪ Enlarged Breasts in Men ▪ Extra Breasts ▪ Triple Nipples ▪ Inverted Nipples ▪ Crusty Nipples ▪ Leaky Nipples ▪ Apple-Shaped Body ▪ Sudden or Unexplained Weight Change ▪ Shrinking ▪ Curved Back ▪ Hunched Back ▪ Unsteadiness ▪ Stiff, Rigid Gait ▪ Double-Jointedness ▪ Stiff Joints ▪ Creaky Knees ▪ Being Left-Handed ▪ Knobby Knuckles ▪ Club-Like Fingers ▪ Curled Fingers ▪ Bump on the Wrist or Hand ▪ Twisted Toes ▪ A Bump on Your Heel ▪ Body Tingling and Numbness ▪ Numb or Tingly Extremities ▪ That Funny-Bone Feeling ▪ Tingly, Numb Fingers ▪ Tingly, Numb Feet ▪ Night Jerks ▪ Jittery Legs ▪ Leg Cramps During the Night ▪ Leg Cramps During the Day ▪ Tremors ▪ Feeling Your Heart Beat ▪ Cold Hands and Feet ▪ Feeling Cold All Over ▪ Feeling Hot When It's Not

CHAPTER 8. PRIVATE PARTS, FARTS, AND BODY WASTES   195

Crooked Penis ▪ A Prolonged Erection ▪ Spotted Penis ▪ Scrotal Swelling ▪ A Swollen Penis Head ▪ A Lump on the Testicle ▪ Red Ejaculate ▪ Penile Discharge ▪ Vaginal Farts ▪ Vaginal Discharge ▪ A Gurgling Stomach ▪ Excessive Burping ▪ Frequent Farting ▪ Feeling Bloated ▪ Green Stools ▪ Orange Stools ▪ Red or Maroon Stools ▪ Black, Tarry Stools ▪ Pale Poop ▪ Floating Feces ▪ Greasy, Smelly Stools ▪ Slimy Stools ▪ Skinny Stools ▪ Colored Urine ▪ Smelly Urine ▪ Sweet Pee ▪ Foamy Urine ▪ Cloudy Urine ▪ Frequent Urination ▪ Leaking Urine ▪ Profuse Perspiration ▪ Night Sweats ▪ No Sweat ▪ Smelly Sweat

CHAPTER 9. SCRATCHING THE SURFACE: YOUR NAILS AND SKIN 239

INTRODUCTION

We all notice things about our bodies that are annoying, weird, unsightly, or downright embarrassing. Our nails may be yellow. Skin tags may suddenly pop up under our breasts. Or our partners may complain that we smell like ammonia. These are body signs. If we learn how to decode them, they can tell us a lot about our state of health . . . or illness.

Fortunately, many body signs are often benign. By this we mean an indicator of a condition that is harmless or medically unimportant. (This use of the word should not be confused with *benign* as the opposite of *malignant* or *cancerous*.) Body signs that are benign can simply be ignored or treated cosmetically. But some body signs may signal something more serious. While those yellowed nails may be nicotine stains, they may also be a warning sign of a lung or liver disorder. Unsightly skin tags—a common sign of aging—may signal diabetes. And while the ammonia-like odor you give off may mean you should hire a cleaning service, it can also mean that you're eating too much protein. Or it may be a warning sign that you're harboring the *Helicobacter pylori* bacterium, the bug that causes stomach ulcers. These medical messages are not merely random occurrences. Rather, they are sent by our bodies to warn us that something may be out of kilter.

Body Signs is about how our bodies communicate our internal health status through external signs and signals. Unlike symptoms, which tend to involve pain or discomfort and are likely to send you running to your doctor's office or even the emergency room, body signs are more likely to send you scurrying off to your hairdresser, nail salon, cosmetic counter, or drugstore. Or if you do go to a doctor, you're more apt to consult a plastic surgeon than an internist. But an internist may be exactly what you need. Sometimes what may seem like a cosmetic concern is more than meets the eye. For example, small, yellowish, and often ugly skin growths may show up on your eyelids. Medically known as *xanthelasmas,* they're actually tiny deposits of cholesterol forewarning that you may have high cholesterol and be at risk for heart disease.

WHAT'S THE DIFFERENCE BETWEEN A BODY SIGN AND A SYMPTOM?

Symptoms—such as pain, fever, and bleeding—come in loud and clear. But body signs tend to be more subtle and difficult to interpret; we may find them dull and banal, embarrassing and bizarre, or anything in between. As John Brown, a 19th-century Scottish physician, put it, "Symptoms are the body's mother tongue; signs are in a foreign language." And while only patients can describe their symptoms, many body signs can be detected by patients, physicians, partners, and even passersby. Body signs are detected by using the five senses; they can be seen, heard, tasted, felt, or smelled.

WHAT CAN OUR BODY SIGNS TELL US?

Before modern diagnostic techniques, doctors had to rely on what their own and their patients' five senses revealed to them. For centuries physicians listened to patients' hearts, felt their pulses, looked at their tongues, eyeballed their eyes, inspected their hair, skin, and nails, smelled their smells, studied their stools, sniffed and sometimes even tasted their urine. Doctors today, even though they usually have sophisticated diagnostic equipment at their disposal, still apply these sensible techniques— with the possible exception of tasting urine.

A good diagnostician has to be an efficient and effective detective. To diagnose even a simple disease, a doctor has to collect countless clues to put together all the pieces of the puzzle so that they cohere into a whole picture. Our visible body parts, especially our hair, eyes, teeth, skin, and nails, can be read as evidence of diseases and disorders that are progressing deep beneath the surface. Sorting through the multitude of signs requires a great deal of detective work and often more than one detective. That's where you—and *Body Signs*—come in.

WHAT *BODY SIGNS* COVERS

Body Signs explores a myriad of signs, some benign, some bad, and some merely bizarre. It covers everything from the head and shoulders to the knees and toes and everything in between. Here are just some of the body signs that may—or may not—spell trouble:

- Striped hair
- Hairy tongue
- Metallic taste
- Eye flashes
- Inverted nipples
- Moonless nails
- Floating stools

Starting at the top, *Body Signs* combs through such hair signs as changes in texture, prematurely gray hair, and unusual hair loss. From there, we head for the head. Not only does the head house our brain, but it's the exclusive home of four of our five senses and the parts that house them—our eyes, ears, nose, and mouth.

Because so much of our self-image is based on our facial features, we tend to focus excessively, if not obsessively, on face-based signs. Though looking at yellow eyes, red noses, and blue lips may horrify us, we shouldn't turn away, because these unattractive anomalies may reveal important clues to serious underlying conditions, such as liver or lung disease.

While the head contains the brain, the torso holds all of our other vital organs: the heart, stomach, liver, kidneys, breasts, and reproductive system. These body parts produce many subtle and easily ignored body signs that can sometimes signal serious disorders.

Chronic hiccups, for example, may be a sign of drinking too much— or an early warning sign of tumors in the esophagus. Excessive flatulence can be caused by a love of raw onions—or may be a sign of gallstones. Urine that smells like overripe apples could be the result of drinking too much apple cider—or a sign of a faulty metabolism. If we close our eyes, shut our ears, and turn up our noses at the often embarrassing signs related to our bodily functions, we may be missing critical clues about our health habits or our health status.

Body Signs also tackles our arms, legs, fingers, and toes. These limbs and digits are our most physically used body parts and, therefore, get the most wear and tear. No wonder they often develop unsightly or bothersome signs such as crooked fingers or creaky knees, to name but a few. But crooked fingers can signal **Dupuytren's disease,** a rare, slowly progressing, debilitating disorder; and creaky knees can be an early sign of *osteoarthritis,* another potentially disabling condition. Finger- and toenails also take a lot of abuse from both inside and out. Cracked nails, for example, can be caused by using household cleaners without gloves—or by nutritional deficiencies.

Body Signs wraps up with the skin. Our skin, the body's largest organ and its most visible and vulnerable, can display a mass of signs: bumps, lumps, freckles, moles, liver spots, spider veins, wrinkles, and dimples. Its color, texture, and tone can all be important clues to countless diseases hidden beneath its surface. While many skin signs are merely cosmetic concerns, some may signify nutritional or hormonal problems, or—most important—cancer.

WHAT *BODY SIGNS* DOES *NOT* COVER

Body Signs is for adults; it does not cover body signs that primarily affect children. And for the most part, it doesn't cover bleeding, fever, fainting, vomiting, pain, or pus. Nor does it cover extreme or chronic itchiness, fatigue, weakness, dizziness, or psychological signs. These are signs and symptoms that should send you running to your doctor or even the emergency room. Finally, *Body Signs* doesn't cover diagnostic tests or treatments. That's strictly between you and your doctor—and all too often your insurance company.

WHAT *BODY SIGNS* CAN AND CAN'T DO

Body Signs is not meant to be a substitute for seeking medical advice and talking with your doctor. On the contrary, it should be a catalyst for communicating with your doctor about things you may not have thought of discussing or might have been too embarrassed to bring up. And *Body Signs* is certainly not meant to turn you into your own doctor. It is, however, intended to help you interpret your body's sign language of sickness and wellness and learn which signs can be safely disregarded and which warrant medical attention.

Body Signs will clue you in on how to be your own diagnostic detective, sniffing out hidden health clues to bring to the attention of your physician. It will enable you to actively participate in your health care as an equal partner with your doctor. By becoming a good diagnostic detective, you can help your doctor determine what's wrong with you when you're sick. Diagnosis is a puzzle, literally and figuratively. To make an accurate diagnosis, your doctor needs all the pieces of the puzzle. Anything you can do to speed up the diagnostic process is helpful. And you hold the puzzle pieces in your hand...and other body parts.

While *Body Signs* is meant to alert you, warn you, and maybe even scare you into going to the doctor, it's also meant to reassure you. Many of the body signs that may concern you will turn out to be perfectly normal and benign. And learning that a sign is normal can save you the time, expense, and anxiety of going to a doctor.

We also hope to both educate and entertain you. *Body Signs* is replete with interesting facts, quotes, and historical anecdotes about the human body.

HOW TO USE *BODY SIGNS*

Body Signs does not have to be read from front to back, nor from head to toe (or hair to toenail, to be more precise). Of course, if you want to, go right ahead. Most people will gravitate toward the body part and the sign that most concerns or interests them. But we can guarantee that in each chapter you'll find something surprising and interesting. It may be a sign you hadn't thought about or realized had medical importance, or information about how your body works—and breaks down. And even if you don't have a specific sign now, *Body Signs* will alert you to signs that may pop up in the future—something to be on the lookout for.

Even if a sign doesn't apply to you, it might be of significance to someone near and dear to you. Indeed, *Body Signs* will help you become a diagnostic detective for your partner, parents, adult children, co-workers, friends, and even foes. For example, if your husband—who's always seen life through rose-colored glasses—starts complaining that things are looking blue, it may not be because he's depressed. Rather, it may be a sign that he's having an undesirable reaction to Viagra.

In addition to descriptions of the signs and what they signify, you will find many *Signposts* scattered throughout each chapter, each one with its own specific icon. Here are examples of the seven different types of *Signposts*.

HEALTHY SIGNS: Signs that are normal and can safely be ignored.

Healthy Sign
Healthy urine is either clear or slightly yellow, and not foamy or frothy.

WARNING SIGNS: Signs that may require medical attention and should be mentioned to your doctor.

Warning Sign
If you constantly crave salt and salty foods, it may be an early warning sign of Addison's disease, a serious autoimmune disease affecting the adrenal glands.

DANGER SIGNS: Signs that require immediate medical attention.

Danger Sign
An increase in flashes—or flashes along with floaters—can be a sign of a retinal tear, a retinal detachment, or an acute vitreous detachment, all of which require immediate medical attention. Even when these conditions are treated, the flashes may persist for several months.

SIGN OF THE TIMES: Historical anecdotes about the human body and its body signs.

Sign of the Times
Ancient Egyptians used borax, duck grease, and cow's milk to treat middle-ear infections. Human breast milk was Hippocrates's drug of choice. He also advised his patients to drink sweet wine and avoid the sun, wind, and smoke-filled rooms.

SPEAKING OF SIGNS: Quotations or sayings related to body signs.

Speaking of Signs
Middle age is when your old classmates are so gray and
wrinkled and bald they don't recognize you.

—Bennett Cerf, 20th-century American author
and co-founder of Random House

SIGNIFICANT FACTS: Little-known, often weird, and occasionally useful facts or stats about various body parts or signs.

Significant Fact
People of European and African descent usually have wet, sticky, brown earwax; those of Native American and Asian descent tend to have dry, brittle, gray, or beige earwax. Women with wet earwax appear to be at increased risk for breast cancer. Indeed, Japanese women with European-like wet earwax have a higher rate of breast cancer than Japanese women with Asian-type dry earwax.

STOP SIGNS: Strategies for preventing signs from occurring or recurring.

Stop Sign
Wearing sunglasses whenever you're out in the sun not only helps protect your eyes from cataracts and skin cancer, but also helps prevent dark circles under the eyes.

SIGNING OFF: This section will appear at the end of each chapter. It will reiterate what types of signs are not covered in the chapter (i.e., pain and bleeding) and list the specialists who are trained to diagnose and treat the medical problems relevant to the key body parts and signs in that particular chapter. When we refer to doctors, we mean both medical doctors (MDs) and doctors

of osteopathic medicine (DOs), who have similar medical training. We sometimes list other health care providers who, while not
physicians, go through special training.

Body Signs also contains several important appendices. These include:

- APPENDIX I: *Body Signs Review: Multisystem Diseases and
  their Signs.* Because so many diseases and disorders have multiple body signs, we've put together a list of some of the most frequently mentioned illnesses and their most common signs.
- APPENDIX II: *Body of Resources: Recommended Websites and
  Books.* A list of reliable medical resources on the Internet and a
  list of books that look at the body from a historical or social per-
  spective.
- APPENDIX III: *My Body Signs Checkup Checklist.* These
  blank charts will help you keep track of your body signs—how
  they look, feel, smell, sound, or taste, and when you first noticed
  them. Because many body signs are reactions to both prescription and over-the-counter drugs (including vitamins and herbal
  supplements), there's also a section to list what medications
  you've been taking and the dosage of each. This chart can be a
  wonderful diagnostic tool, one you can bring to your doctor so he
  or she can have a better sense of what you've been experiencing.

WHY WE WROTE THIS BOOK

One of us, Joan Liebmann-Smith, became interested in body signs more
than twenty years ago when she ignored some serious signs that should
have sent her running to her doctor. Rather, she wrote most of them off
as annoyances she ascribed to being a new mom. She was hot and sweaty
all the time, but she blamed that on having turned up the thermostat to
keep her newborn warm. She was also losing sleep, losing hair, and losing weight (which she considered a good sign)—all signs she attributed
to nursing her fussy baby around the clock.

Luckily, she had lunch one day with a perceptive relative who, upon seeing her, blurted out, "You have a goiter!" Stunned, Joan darted into the ladies' room and looked in the mirror. Sure enough, there it was: a lump the size of a lemon on her neck—something not only she but also her husband and numerous physician friends had neglected to notice.

When she saw her doctor the next day, he told her she had a very advanced case of Graves' disease, the most common form of hyperthyroidism. Her body, he said, was literally eating itself up, and all those body signs she had disregarded were, in fact, classic signs of the disease. Without immediate treatment—which involved taking radioactive iodine—she most likely would have been dead within a week. Joan had to wean her baby the next day and leave home for several days after the treatment, because she was going to be temporarily radioactive.

Had she read a book like *Body Signs,* she would have spared herself—and her husband and baby—the physical and emotional crisis they experienced. She certainly would have paid more attention to the warning signs and seen her doctor sooner, thus avoiding having an easily detectable and highly treatable condition turn into a truly grave and life-threatening illness.

When Joan mentioned that she was planning to write *Body Signs* to Jacqueline Egan, her friend, colleague, and co-author of two of her books, Jacqueline's interest was immediately piqued. As a medical writer, recent widow, and cancer survivor, Jacqueline was keenly aware of the importance of early detection. When she was thirty-five, she noticed a small lump in her breast. Luckily, that growth turned out not to be cancer, as was also the case with several others she found during the next fifteen years. But she remained extremely watchful and cautious. In 2001, three months after her husband Ed's untimely death from a heart attack, she kept an appointment for a mammogram and a malignant growth was found.

Jacqueline credits vigilance with saving her life. But her closest friend, Corinne, was not as fortunate. She and her doctors missed a subtle sign of ovarian cancer—abdominal bloating. Sad to say, Corinne died during the writing of this book.

Joan and Jacqueline wrote *Body Signs* to help you avoid similar ordeals by alerting you to the warning signs of potentially dangerous disorders and diseases. We don't want to scare you—we just want to help you become good diagnostic detectives, adept at detecting and decoding the signs your body is sending you.

BODY SIGNS PANEL OF MEDICAL EXPERTS

Pete S. Batra, MD
Assistant Professor of Surgery
Section of Nasal and Sinus Disorders
Head and Neck Institute
Cleveland Clinic
Cleveland, Ohio

Wilma Bergfeld, MD
Section Head of Clinical Research
Section Department of Dermatology
Cleveland Clinic
Cleveland, Ohio

Michael L. Bloom, DDS
Attending
Lenox Hill Hospital
New York, New York

Stephen J. DiMartino, MD, PhD
Assistant Attending Physician
Hospital for Special Surgery/
    New York Presbyterian Hospital
Instructor of Clinical Medicine
Weill Cornell Medical College
New York, New York

Loren Wissner Greene, MD
Clinical Associate Professor
Department of Medicine
Co-director, Osteoporosis and
    Metabolic Bone Disease Program
    of the Department of Medicine
New York University School of
    Medicine
New York, New York

Axel Grothey, MD
Senior Associate Consultant
Division of Medical Oncology
Mayo Clinic
Rochester, Minnesota

Stuart I. Henochowicz, MD
Associate Clinical Professor
Division of Allergy, Immunology,
   and Rheumatology
Georgetown University Medical
   School
Washington, DC

Gordon Hughes, MD
Professor and Head
Head of Otology and Neurotology
Head and Neck Institute
Cleveland Clinic
Cleveland, Ohio

Alan Kominsky, MD
Vice Chairman
Head and Neck Institute
Cleveland Clinic
Cleveland, Ohio

Ronald B. Kraft, MD
Assistant Professor of Clinical
   Medicine
Weill Cornell Medical Center
New York, New York

Sharon Lewin, MD
Assistant Clinical Professor of
   Medicine

Columbia University, College of
   Physicians and Surgeons
New York, New York

Larry Lipshultz, MD
Professor, Scott Department of
   Urology
Baylor College of Medicine
Houston, Texas

Michael Osborne, MD
Director
Breast Cancer Programs of
   Continuum Cancer Centers of
   New York
New York, New York

Rochelle L. Peck, MD
Attending Physician
Montefiore Medical Center
St. Luke's-Roosevelt Medical
   Center
Clinical Instructor, Department of
   Ophthalmology
Columbia University, College of
   Physicians and Surgeons
New York, New York

Rock Positano, DPM, MSc, MPH
Director
Non-surgical Foot and Ankle
   Service
Hospital for Special Surgery
New York Presbyterian Hospital
New York, New York

Joseph Scharpf, MD
Associate
Head and Neck Institute
Cleveland Clinic
Cleveland, Ohio

John J. Stangel, MD
Medical Director
Westchester County
Reproductive Medicine Associates
  of Connecticut

The Center for Advanced
  Reproductive Medicine
Norwalk, Connecticut

Randall M. Zusman, MD
Associate Professor of Medicine
Harvard Medical School
Director, Division of Hypertension
  and Vascular Medicine
Massachusetts General Hospital
Boston, Massachusetts

DISCLAIMER: The *Body Signs* Panel of Medical Experts list their affiliations for informational purposes only. The listed affiliations do not imply endorsement of this book by those medical institutions.

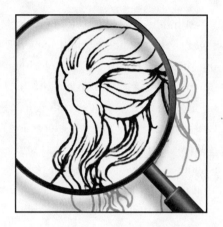

CHAPTER 1

YOUR HAIR

The Long and the Short of It

Gimme a head with hair,
   long beautiful hair
Shining, gleaming, steaming,
   flaxen, waxen
Give me down to there, hair!
Shoulder length or longer . . .
   hair!

—"HAIR," 1968

Hair defines us like no other part of the human body. It conveys to others an enormous amount of information: our age, gender, ethnicity, social status, religious and other group affiliations, personal hygiene habits, and—last but not least—our state of health. Yet the assumptions some people make based on our hair may be as false as their eyelashes. We can cover the gray, making us appear years younger; cut our hair very short or let it grow very long, making it difficult to determine our gender; or straighten curly hair or curl straight hair, making our ethnicity anyone's guess. And by adopting the hairstyles of the rich and famous, we can look like we're to the manor born when we may be struggling to make (split) ends meet.

Hair is overflowing with sexual symbolism and cultural significance.

People in many parts of the world routinely—if not religiously—cover or remove it. English barristers, for example, wear wigs in court. Muslim and Orthodox Jewish women are required to cover their heads. And not only do Buddhists and some Christian monks shave their heads, but skinheads do as well.

SPEAKING OF SIGNS

The hair is the richest ornament of women.

—Martin Luther,
16th-century German theologian

While we're busy sending messages to the outside world by covering, cropping, curling, or coloring our hair, we should also pay attention to the messages it's sending us. Our untouched, natural hair can give us a headful of vital information that we should carefully read and heed. Your age, sex, and race, as well as where you live and the hair products you use, all affect your hair's mineral makeup.

SIGN OF THE TIMES

In ancient Egypt, both men and women shaved their heads and wore wigs. Priests, however, had to remove each and every hair from their bodies, including their eyebrows and eyelashes.

Hair contains a myriad of minerals, from aluminum to zinc, and for many years hair analysis has been used to confirm mercury and arsenic poisoning. More recently, researchers have been able to diagnose eating disorders from hair samples.

Indeed, the quality, quantity, and color of our hair can all be signs of our physical well-being. No wonder hair is said to be a barometer of health.

STARTING AT THE TOP

HAIR TEXTURE CHANGES

Hair is made up mostly of dead protein (*keratin*), but that doesn't mean it's supposed to lie there listlessly. Dry, brittle hair and split ends can all be signs that you're mistreating your hair with excessive washing, brushing, drying, dyeing, or bleaching. However, these *hair shaft disorders,* as

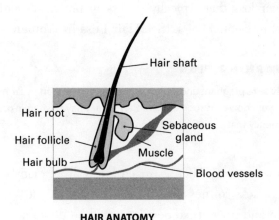

HAIR ANATOMY

they're called, can also be signs of stress, hormonal changes, nutritional deficiencies, and thyroid disease.

If you notice, for example, that your formerly luxuriant locks tangle easily or have become dry, brittle, or coarse, don't be so quick to rush off and buy the latest expensive new hair product. You may, in fact, have the classic signs of *hypothyroidism*—a fairly common but often underdiagnosed condition, especially among women. (See Appendix I.) When the thyroid gland, which regulates metabolism, fails to produce enough thyroid hormone, hair growth—as well as other body functions—slows down. Hair texture change can signal *iodine deficiency* as well, which is also implicated in thyroid disease. (See Chapter 6.)

Of course, texture changes may merely be an indicator of the natural hormone changes of pregnancy or menopause. During pregnancy, dry hair may become oilier or shinier, while oily hair can become drier and duller. Previously curly hair may become straighter and straight hair curlier. Hair may even become thicker, but this is due to the slowing down

SIGNIFICANT FACT

Americans spend almost $10 million each year on hair analysis to help uncover their health and nutritional status.

SIGNIFICANT FACT

Even a single hair is very strong. One reason is that it's made up of the protein keratin, which is highly resistant to wear and tear. Keratin is the same resilient substance found in animal feathers, claws, nails, and hoofs.

of normal hair loss that typically occurs in pregnancy rather than the thickening of individual hairs. (See **Hair Loss in Women,** below.)

WARNING SIGN

If you're pregnant and your hair seems thinner than usual, mention this to your doctor as soon as possible. You may have a vitamin or mineral deficiency that can affect the pregnancy.

During menopause, when estrogen levels drop, many women notice that their hair lacks softness and luster. The estrogen loss can cause hair shafts to thin and dry out, so new hairs will be duller and less manageable. New hair growth also tapers off.

SIGNIFICANT FACT

Your hairdresser can be your friend in more ways than one. Hairdressers are often the first to recognize and remark on hair texture changes. These changes may be the early clues to thyroid conditions and other underdiagnosed disorders.

Both hair texture change and hair loss are also common reactions to chemotherapy or radiation treatment for cancer. The good news is that both these changes are usually temporary.

HAIR COLOR CHANGES

Hair color, like eye and skin color, depends primarily on how much *melanin* (color-producing pigments) we inherit from our parents.

SPEAKING OF SIGNS

I'm not offended by all the dumb-blond jokes because I know that I'm not dumb. I also know I'm not a blond.

—Dolly Parton, country-and-western singer

If your hair color changes and you haven't been hitting the bleach or hair dye bottle, it can be a sign of a variety of factors, both internal and external. For example, hair color—like hair texture—can change temporarily after chemotherapy. A blonde may become dismayed to find her hair growing in dark brown or black, while a former brunette may be thrilled to find that she's become a blonde. Hair color changes can also signal genetic, metabolic, nutritional, or other disorders. They can even be the result of environmental factors.

Green Hair

Many of us look forward to our hair getting lighter from the summer sun. But if your hair looks more green than platinum, it's not the sun's fault. It's more likely to be a tip-off that your swimming pool is heavily chlorinated, or that copper from water pipes is seeping into your pool water. In fact, green hair used to be fairly common among copper- and brassworkers.

STOP SIGN

Rinsing your hair with lemon juice or vinegar may help restore green hair to its natural color.

If you haven't been swimming lately, your sea-green hair can be a sign that you enjoy bathing in a tub that's been cleaned with chlorine-containing products. If your green hair doesn't seem related to swimming or bathing, it could be a more serious sign of excess exposure to mercury, which can cause neurological, muscular, sensory, and cognitive damage.

SIGNIFICANT FACT

Most adults have 100,000 to 150,000 hairs on their scalp at any one time. On average, natural blondes have the most hairs (140,000), while redheads have the fewest (90,000).

Striped Hair

Green hair may be medically unimportant, but striped hair is not. Known as the *flag sign*, the striped hair is actually bands of discolored or depigmented hair. The stripes—usually blond, gray, or reddish—are often red flags for severe nutritional deficiencies, for example, of protein or iron. Although much more common in underdeveloped countries, the flag sign can be seen in children living in poverty throughout the world.

Striped hair can also signal *ulcerative colitis* or other conditions or events that deplete protein, such as *irritable bowel syndrome* (see Chapter 8) or extensive bowel surgery. It might also be a telltale sign of the eating disorder *anorexia nervosa,* which depletes a person's protein supply.

Prematurely Gray Hair

When most people's hair turns gray, it's usually a normal—albeit not very welcome—sign of aging. As we age, we produce less melanin, the pigment that gives our hair and skin its color. But when your hair turns gray before its time, it can be a harmless, hereditary condition—or a warning sign that something is wrong. The definition of premature graying—medically known as *canities*—varies among doctors. Some define it as having half a head of gray hair by age 40; others say it's the graying of hair before the age of 20 in whites and before 30 in blacks.

> **SIGNIFICANT FACT**
>
> Hair is the second-fastest-growing tissue in the body. Bone marrow holds the top place.

Some people with prematurely gray hair may unknowingly suffer from *pernicious anemia,* a severe form of anemia in which there is a reduction of red blood cells caused by the body's inability to absorb vitamin B_{12}. Pernicious anemia is commonly found in older adults. Other common signs of pernicious anemia include paleness, weakness, mouth and tongue problems, tingling and numbness in hands and feet, and an unsteady gait. If untreated, it can cause serious gastrointestinal or neurological problems. The good news is that not only is it treated easily, but hair often returns to its natural color.

> **SIGNIFICANT FACT**
>
> Whites tend to start graying in their mid-30s, Asians in their late 30s, and blacks in their mid-40s. Men usually turn gray before women do.

Early graying can also signal various autoimmune disorders, including Graves' disease, the most common form of hyperthyroidism (see Appendix I). A recent Irish study has identified prematurely gray hair as a sign of low bone mineral density (*osteopenia*) in women with Graves' disease. Another autoimmune disorder signaled by premature graying, as well as by white patches on the skin, is *vitiligo* (see Chapter 9), which is a benign condition. However, 1 in 3 people with vitiligo also suffers from thyroid disease.

Another autoimmune condition, *alopecia areata*, which is characterized by patchy hair loss, is sometimes spotted in young people with gray hair. (See **Spotty or Patchy Hair Loss**, below.)

There is also some disquieting new evidence that prematurely gray hair can be an early warning sign of *diabetes, coronary heart disease* (*CHD*), and an increased risk of heart attack (*myocardial infarction*).

SIGNIFICANT FACT

Hair color changes, including prematurely gray hair, are not always permanent. The hair sometimes reverts to its original color when an underlying condition is treated or after finishing a course of chemotherapy or radiation. But it's not the individual hairs that return to their previous color. Rather, the new hair grows in the original color, and sometimes even darker. So the change will take a while to occur.

WARNING SIGN

Smoking appears linked to hair loss and gray hair. The toxic elements in tobacco smoke can damage the DNA in our hair follicles, as well as the tiny blood vessels nourishing our hair and skin. These and other mechanisms speed up the premature aging process.

Many people think having prematurely gray hair is a sign of stress, and there's some truth to this. One theory is that stress can precipitate autoimmune diseases or the other conditions mentioned above that can cause graying.

WARNING SIGN

A combination of gray hair and dark eyebrows can be striking or sexy (think Sean Connery). But men with this color combo are at high risk for diabetes, according to a recent German study.

Hair Turning White Overnight

While stress may play a role in turning your hair gray, it can't do it overnight. Marie Antoinette's and Sir Thomas More's hair were said to have turned completely white the night before they were beheaded. Despite these and other historical anecdotes, no medical evidence exists that hair can turn white or gray so quickly. Once hair is produced in the hair follicles, individual hairs can't change color. The root of these anecdotes may be *diffuse alopecia areata,* a condition that is sometimes triggered by stress and causes a lot of hair to fall out very quickly. (See **Hair Shedding,** below.) If a person with a mixture of gray and pigmented hairs has this condition, the pigmented hairs are the most likely to be shed, leaving behind only the gray or white hair.

SPEAKING OF SIGNS

Middle age is when your old classmates are so gray and wrinkled and bald they don't recognize you.

—Bennett Cerf, 20th-century American author and co-founder of Random House

LOSING IT

Our head hair grows about half an inch per month. About 90% of our hair is in this growing (*anagen*) phase at any one time, which can last from two to six years. The rest is in the resting (*telogen*) phase, which lasts about two to three months. Then it falls out. On average, our scalps drop about 50 to 100 hairs each day. The exact number usually depends on factors we can't control—heredity, age, gender, and ethnicity. Whether it falls out in clumps or gradually, most of us will experience some hair loss over the course of our lifetimes. By age 50, more than half of women

HEALTHY SIGN

If you *don't* have gray hair, you may both look younger and live longer. A large Danish study found that adult men who did not have gray hair had slightly lower death rates than men with gray hair.

will have lost some locks. But the news is even worse for men. Fully 75% will have lost some hair, and 25% will be bald by that same age.

WARNING SIGN

If you're a man taking the hair restoration drug finasteride (Propecia), be sure to mention it to your doctor before having the PSA screening test for prostate cancer. The drug can interfere with the accuracy of the test results.

SPOTTY OR PATCHY HAIR LOSS

If you notice patches of hair missing from your head, it may be a sign of *alopecia areata*. This is an autoimmune disorder in which the body's white blood cells attack the hair follicles, causing them to stop growing hair. But it's not just scalp hair that can be affected.

Some people lose hair all over their bodies—a condition medically known as *alopecia universalis.* Some mild forms of the different types of alopecia are amenable to treatment. And sometimes the hair even regrows without any outside help. The bad news is that people with alopecia often have or may develop other autoimmune diseases, especially thyroid disease, diabetes, and rheumatoid arthritis.

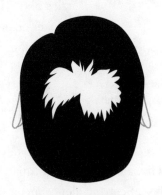

ALOPECIA AREATA

Patches of missing hair can also signal *trichotillomania,* in which people compulsively pull out their head hair or even their eyelashes. This behavioral condition, which is found in 3 to 5% of the U.S. population, is more likely to affect children than adults, but it can occur at any age. It's occasionally mistaken for alopecia areata, but the distinguishing sign of trichotillomania is broken hairs, often of differing lengths. Some hairs also remain in the bald spots. People with this condition often display signs of psychological problems, including depression, anxiety, obsessive-compulsive behavior, and *Tourette syndrome*, a neurological disorder that usually starts in childhood and has the hallmark signs of motor and vocal tics. Trichotillomania occasionally runs in families. Indeed, researchers recently found two mutated genes that may be responsible in some cases.

SPEAKING OF SIGNS

Gray hair is a sign of age, not of wisdom.

—Greek proverb

Gray hair is a crown of glory. It is attained by a life of righteousness.

—Proverbs 16:31

Gray hairs are death's blossoms.

—English proverb

If you have spotty hair loss, your body may also be sending you a strong message that you're overtreating, overbrushing, or overdyeing your hair. Loss of hair because of this is medically known as *traumatic alopecia*. This is a good example of why you should *not* listen to old wives' tales about brushing your hair 100 strokes a day. Although your hair may shine more, it may also fall out! Sporting tight ponytails, cornrows, or braids can cause hair breakage and loss as well.

SPEAKING OF SIGNS

My hair is gray, but not with years,
Nor grew it white
In a single night.
As men's have grown from sudden fears.

—Lord Byron, *The Prisoner of Chillon,* 1816

Spotty hair loss may signal a condition called *cicatricial* or *scarring alopecia,* in which the follicles are destroyed and replaced by scar tissue. Unfortunately, hair won't grow back with this type of hair loss. Scarring alopecia can be the result of a burn, a physical injury, or anything that can cause a scar elsewhere on the body. It can also be a sign of bacterial and fungal infections—including the dreaded *ringworm*—and various other skin diseases, such as *discoid lupus erythematosus*, an autoimmune disorder primarily affecting young women. Unlike the more common (systemic) form of lupus (see Chapter 9 and Appendix I), which involves many parts of the body, discoid lupus affects only the skin, resulting in scarring and hair loss.

BALDING IN MEN

If you're a young man and going bald, you may freak out, fearing that you're losing your virility along with your locks. But your balding head is more likely just an unwelcome legacy from a long line of shiny-pated men on either your father's *or* mother's side. *Male-pattern baldness*, medically known as *androgenetic alopecia*, is nothing to worry about, at least medically. It's a genetic condition caused by excess androgens. (Women also have androgens but in lesser amounts.)

SIGNIFICANT FACT

Japanese men are less likely to become bald than white men. And those who do go bald tend to lose their hair about 10 years later than white men.

However, a recent study of men in their mid-forties with male-pattern baldness found that those with frontal baldness had a slightly increased chance of developing coronary heart disease (CHD) compared with men with no hair loss. Those with hairless crowns (known as *vertex baldness*) were significantly more likely than their hairy counterparts to develop CHD.

SPEAKING OF SIGNS

It is foolish to tear one's hair in grief, as though sorrow would be made less with baldness.

—Cicero, ancient Roman orator and politician

The bigger the bald spot, the bigger the risk. Men who were bald on top and also had high cholesterol or high blood pressure were at highest risk.

HAIR LOSS IN WOMEN

When you part your hair, does it remind you of the parting of the Red Sea? Seeing your scalp shining through can be a sign of *female-pattern baldness*. Like male-pattern baldness, it is medically known as *androgenetic alopecia* and can be inherited from either parent. Because of the connec-

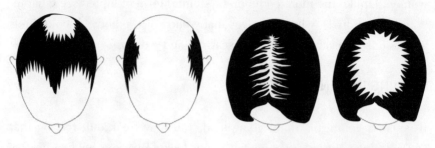

MALE-PATTERN BALDNESS   **FEMALE-PATTERN BALDNESS**

tion to androgens, female-pattern baldness can be the first warning sign of a type of diabetes that's related to excess androgens.

However, the pattern of balding in women is different than in men. Women are more likely to have thinning head hair rather than the completely bald patches or receding hairlines that are the hallmarks of male-pattern baldness.

Hair loss in women can also be a normal sign of aging and hormonal changes, especially after childbirth and during menopause. Many women experience hair loss a few months after they stop taking birth control pills or hormone replacement therapy. Interestingly, hair loss slows and hair growth accelerates during pregnancy. The result: a fuller- and thicker-looking head of hair. Unfortunately, this windfall doesn't last; three to four months after a woman gives birth, the extra hairs shed rapidly. The good news is that hair growth will return to normal and the new moms will once again have full heads of hair, probably by the time their babies do.

> ### SPEAKING OF SIGNS
>
> *I told you to stop using rinses—and now just look at you!*
> *No hair worth mentioning left to dye.*
> *Why couldn't you let it well alone?*
> *If your hair's fallen out, it's not any envious tongue that's to blame.*
> *You applied that concoction yourself. It was you that did it. All your fault....*
>
> —Ovid, ancient Roman poet
> Amores I:14

HAIR SHEDDING

A ton of hair on the shower floor, in your brush, or on your pillow is not a pretty sight. Medically known as ***sudden, diffuse hair loss*** or ***telogen ef-***

fluvium, it's the second most common form of hair loss. (Male-pattern baldness takes top place.) In this condition the hairs in the growing (anagen) phase prematurely go into the resting (telogen) phase. (See **Losing It,** above.) The result: more hairs than usual are cast off. And, as its name implies, the shedding occurs all over the scalp, rather than following a typical pattern of baldness.

Losing lots of hair at once can also be a sign that you've been under a great deal of psychological stress; have suffered some recent physical trauma, such as a car accident or major surgery; or have a skin disorder, such as psoriasis (see Chapter 9) or eczema. The reason for this is unknown.

SIGN OF THE TIMES

The Polish-French composer and pianist Chopin was purported to have had a beard on only the right side of his face—the side seen by the audience. The unseen side, he claimed, didn't matter.

Unfortunately, as most of us are all too aware, sudden hair loss can be a reaction to chemotherapy and radiation treatment for cancer. Just as these treatments stop rapidly dividing cancer cells from multiplying, they also stop the rapidly growing hair cells. The result is that as much as 90% of hair can be lost, usually within the first month of treatment. Happily, about six months to a year after cancer treatment ends, hair generally grows back.

Sudden shedding can also be a delayed sign of a recent high fever

SIGNIFICANT FACT

If you have male-pattern baldness, you're not likely to have the shiny-domed look of Yul Brenner, Michael Jordan, or Bruce Willis unless you shave your head. Male-pattern baldness always leaves a horseshoe-shaped fringe of hair around the scalp, often called a *monk's cap.*

or an indication that you're currently fighting a viral, bacterial, or fungal infection. But in these cases, you're likely to have other signs, such as itching, skin irritation, fever, or pain. It can also be an early warning sign of a hormonal disorder, especially thyroid disease (see Appendix I) or hypopituitarism; indeed, almost any hormonal imbalance can cause hair shedding.

If you've changed your eating habits or have been on a crash diet and you're losing your hair as well as weight, it may be a tip-off that you have a nutritional problem such as an iron, protein, or zinc deficiency. Hair loss may also be a telltale sign that you eat lots of raw eggs—eating too many raw egg whites, or foods containing raw egg whites such as mayonnaise, mousse, steak tartare, or Caesar salad dressing, can lead to a rare condition called *biotin deficiency* (aka *egg-white injury syndrome*). Other early warning signs may include dry skin, rashes, and fine, brittle hair. If untreated, neurological and intestinal problems can develop within weeks. So if you love to eat egg whites, be sure to thoroughly heat them first. You'll be killing two birds with one stone: reducing your risk of egg-white injury syndrome and of salmonella food poisoning.

Nutritional deficiencies aren't the only culprits. Hair loss can also be your body's way of telling you that you've had too much of a good thing. Indeed, an excess of certain medicines or even essential vitamins and minerals (especially *vitamin A* and *selenium*) can cause your hair to fall out.

SIGN OF THE TIMES

High foreheads were considered a sign of beauty in Elizabethan England. Fashionable ladies shaved or plucked their front hairs to achieve this look. They also applied bandages soaked in vinegar and rubbed with cat's dung as a depilatory.

HAIR THAT IS—OR ISN'T—THERE

How much hair we have—and where it is or isn't—depends to a great extent on the roll of the genetic dice. Both hairiness and hairlessness often run in families and among certain ethnic groups. Native American men, for example, tend to have very little, if any, facial hair. And men from East Africa are apt to have a lot more facial hair than their neighbors in West Africa. Chest hair also varies by ethnic background; the hairiest chests are sported by men of Middle Eastern, South Asian, and European descent.

Ethnicity can also be a factor in hair growth in women. Asian and

SIGNIFICANT FACT

Locks of Love (locksoflove.org) is a nonprofit organization that provides wigs and hairpieces to children suffering from hair loss from cancer treatments or other conditions. So if you have 10 or 12 inches of nongray hair to spare, don't just leave it on your hairdresser's floor—donate it to Locks of Love!

Native American women tend to have little body hair, while Middle Eastern and Mediterranean women tend to have considerably more.

BORN (HAIR) FREE

If you're the only man in your family and among your friends who doesn't have to shave and you don't have much chest, pubic, or underarm hair, you may have been born with a chromosomal disorder known as *Klinefelter's syndrome*. This is a relatively rare abnormality. Other typical Klinefelter's signs include being tall, being pear-shaped, having small genitals, and sometimes having enlarged breasts. (See Chapter 7.) But men with this syndrome may either lack these signs or ignore them. Indeed, a man may not know he has it until he and his partner consult a reproductive endocrinologist or other fertility specialist because they're not getting pregnant. Because men with Klinefelter's tend to have abnormally low levels of testosterone and high levels of estrogen, they often suffer from infertility and sexual dysfunction.

SIGNIFICANT FACT

Beards are the fastest-growing hairs on the human body. The average man's beard would grow to almost 30 feet if he never trimmed it.

WARNING SIGN

Men with Klinefelter's syndrome are at increased risk for osteoporosis and some serious autoimmune disorders, such as rheumatoid arthritis and lupus. It also raises their chances of developing breast cancer, testicular cancer, lung disease, and *extragonadal germ cell tumors*, rare growths that can be cancerous.

The good news is that many men with this condition who suffer from infertility may be able to father children with the help of advanced reproductive technologies. And with testosterone treatment, men with Klinefelter's can grow hair and have a better sex life to boot.

LOSING EYEBROWS OR EYELASHES

If you notice that your previously lush lashes or bushy brows are nowhere to be seen, it may be another unfortunate sign of aging.

SPEAKING OF SIGNS

A hairy body, and arms stiff with bristles, give promise of a manly soul.

—Juvenal, ancient Roman poet

But eyelash loss—known medically as *madarosis*—can also be an early warning sign of hyperthyroidism (see **Prematurely Gray Hair,** above) or a tip-off that you're consuming too much vitamin A. And if it's just the hairs of your outer eyebrows that fall out, it may mean that you have *Hashimoto's syndrome,* a chronic form of hypothyroidism. (See Chapter 6.)

MOVIN' ON DOWN

LOSING CHEST AND BODY HAIR

To the ancient Greeks and Romans, a hairless chest on a man was the aesthetic ideal, possibly because it represented youth. Today, however, chest hair on a man is considered a classic sign of masculinity and a source of pride in many cultures. As with head hair, if a man's chest hair starts to go, his ego may not be far behind. Losing chest and body hair can be a normal sign of aging or signal an androgen deficiency, which itself is often related to aging. It may also be a sign of alopecia areata. (See **Spotty or Patchy Hair Loss,** above.)

LOSING PUBIC HAIR

Many of us choose to pluck, shave, wax, burn, or otherwise remove unwanted hair from various parts of our bodies. Indeed, one of the latest crazes among some young women is shaving their pubic hair. But when our pubic hair starts to fall out on its own, it may not be quite the fashion statement we wish to make.

Thinning pubic hair in women is a perfectly natural sign of aging, indicating that estrogen levels are dipping, which happens around menopause. Although men may also lose pubic hair as they age, the loss is usually less obvious.

At any age and in either sex, scanty pubic hair—as well as loss of underarm hair—can be a sign of hypopituitarism (see **Hair Shedding,** above). It may also indicate another serious but rare hormonal disorder, *Addison's disease*, a potentially life-threatening disease that involves the destruction of the adrenal glands and affects the mucous membranes and skin as well as the hair. (See Chapter 9 and Appendix I.)

SIGN OF THE TIMES

In the 16th century, the Russian tsar Ivan the Terrible declared that shaving a beard was a sin. When Peter the Great took over the crown, he believed that a shaved face was a sign of progressiveness; he considered beards archaic and ridiculous. He personally cut off the beards of his noblemen and levied a "beard tax" on men who continued to wear them. Priests and peasants were exempt.

HAIR, THERE, AND EVERYWHERE

HAIR IN ALL THE WRONG PLACES

Bearded ladies have long been fixtures in circuses and amusement-park freak shows. But if a woman notices hairs sprouting from her previously smooth chin or a moustache growing under her very nose, she's probably *not* amused.

Unwelcome facial hair can be a harmless sign of aging. Although many women experience thinning hair or hair loss during menopause (see **Hair Loss in Women,** above), others may notice just the opposite as their estrogen production slows and becomes overshadowed by androgen. Both sexes have androgen and

SIGNIFICANT FACTS

The growing cycle for scalp hair is 2 to 6 years. For eyelashes and eyebrows, it's 1 to 6 months.

estrogen; it's the amount and proportion of each that dictates how much hair we have and where we have it.

Hair growing where it shouldn't and excessive hair growth anywhere are typical signs of having too much androgen. Medically known as *hirsutism*—pronounced "*her*-suit-ism"—it can occur in either sex. While men may not consider it much of a problem, it can be exceedingly embarrassing for women. Unwanted hair in women is often dark and coarse and sprouts in places where men typically have hair—on the chin, chest, lip, thighs, ears, or face, or around the nipples.

SIGN OF THE TIMES

In 2004, Lloyd's of London began offering a unique form of insurance: men could be covered for chest hair loss for up to £1 million.

WARNING SIGN

Lanugo—the fine hair newborns have covering their bodies—is sometimes seen on adults. When it is, it may be a sign of the eating disorder *anorexia nervosa*.

Women with hirsutism may also have a deep voice, big muscles, small breasts, an enlarged clitoris, and irregular periods—all signs of an androgen-related hormone disorder called *masculinization*.

With or without these other signs, hirsutism can be an unfortunate reaction to hormone-containing drugs, such as birth control pills, steroids, fertility drugs, and testosterone. And not surprisingly, excess hair growth can be a side effect of minoxidil (Rogaine), the antihypertensive drug, which is also commonly used as a hair loss treatment. Hirsutism can also be a clue to the overuse or abuse of anabolic steroids.

SIGN OF THE TIMES

In 15th-century England, women shaved their pubic hair to keep lice at bay. They covered up the bare spots with merkins—pubic wigs. Merkins were also popular among prostitutes for another reason: they covered up the telltale signs of syphilis and other venereal diseases.

Excessive facial and body hair in women are often signs of *polycystic ovarian syndrome* (PCOS). Also called *polycystic ovarian disease* (*PCOD*) and *Stein-Leventhal syndrome,* it's one of the most under- or misdiagnosed conditions in women of reproductive age. Other common signs include acne and being overweight. Women with PCOS—which is caused by the overproduction of androgens—have either irregular or missing periods. In fact, PCOS is a leading cause of infertility.

WARNING SIGN

Women with excess androgens from such conditions as PCOS or Cushing's syndrome are at increased risk for uterine cancer, insulin resistance, and high cholesterol levels. PCOS may also be an early warning sign of heart disease.

Hirsutism can signal another kind of hormonal disorder, known as *Cushing's syndrome* or *hypercortisolism.* Rather than being androgen-driven (as in PCOS), the excessive hair growth of Cushing's is due to the adrenal glands producing too much of the stress hormone cortisol. Both women and men can have Cushing's, and it usually strikes between the ages of 20 and 50. Women with Cushing's often have hair on their face, neck, chest, abdomen, and thighs. Other common signs include irregular or missing periods, acne and other skin problems, and weight gain around the midsection and upper back.

SIGNIFICANT FACT

Have you ever wondered why your arm, armpit, chest, leg, and pubic hairs never grow really long? It's because these hairs are in the growing phase for only a few months but remain in the resting phase for years.

WARNING SIGN

If you're plagued by excess hair and acne and are also overly tired and achy, you may have chronic hepatitis or another serious disorder.

Excess hair growth can also signal the presence of ovarian cysts. These fluid-filled growths, which tend to occur during the childbearing years, are usually not cancerous. However, older women with ovarian cysts are at increased risk of developing ovarian cancer. In fact, facial hair in a post-menopausal woman may actually be a red flag for ovarian cancer.

VERY HAIRY MEN

Just like bearded ladies, so-called werewolves have been standard attractions at side shows. This type of excessive hair growth in men, medically known as *congenital hypertrichosis,* is exceedingly rare. However, there is a less severe and more common form of this condition, known as *acquired hypertrichosis,* which can occur as a drug reaction to some topical steroids, antibiotics, drugs to treat epilepsy, and hair growth drugs. Stopping the drug will usually stop the excess hair growth. Excess hair growth in men can also be a sign of a skin disease called *lichen simplex,* which involves thickening of the skin too. (See Chapter 9.) In addition, excessive hair growth in men may signal a metabolic skin condition called *porphyria cutanea tarda,* which also causes blisters to develop on sun-exposed areas. Porphyria cutanea tarda is associated with several liver problems, including hepatitis C, which can lead to cirrhosis or even liver cancer if untreated.

SIGN OF THE TIMES

Vivian Wheeler, who suffered from hirsutism, was forced by her mother to shave her face at the tender age of 7. After her mother died in the early 1990s, she decided it was time to renounce the daily drudgery of shaving. Within a few years, her beard was 11 inches long. She joined a local "oddity" show and even made it into the *Guinness Book of World Records.*

WARNING SIGN

Female relatives of very hairy men may be at risk for PCOS.

SIGNING OFF

Clearly, your hair problem shouldn't necessarily be brushed off as a mere cosmetic concern. While hair loss isn't usually an immediate life-threatening sign, if you see signs of other hair-related conditions, you should gather them up and consult your primary care physician. Most likely, he or she can either resolve the problem or refer you to a specialist who can. The following are specialists trained to diagnose and treat many problems related to the hair and scalp.

- *Dermatologist:* A medical doctor who has been trained in diagnosing and treating skin and hair diseases. (Don't forget, hair is actually skin.)
- *Endocrinologist:* A medical doctor who specializes in evaluating and treating hormone disorders, many of which are responsible for hair problems.

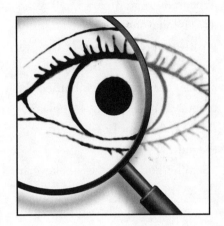

CHAPTER 2

READING YOUR EYES

He speaketh not; and yet
there lies
A conversation in his eyes.

—HENRY WADSWORTH LONGFELLOW,
"THE HANGING OF THE CRANE," 1875

Our eyes—with more than two million working parts—are the second most complex organ in our bodies. (The brain takes first place.) Their primary function, sight, is considered by many to be the most important of our senses. But the significance of eyes goes well beyond their physiological role.

Since ancient times, eyes have been a source of both fascination and fear. Their ability to mesmerize those who gaze into them reinforced the widespread belief that eyes are powerful sources of evil. Indeed, this fear of the "evil eye" and its ability to harm children, adults, livestock, and even crops is one of the most ancient and universal superstitions. References to the evil eye can be seen scattered throughout the Talmud, the Bible, and the Koran. Belief in the evil eye, called *mal occhio* by the Italians, *mal de ojo* by the Spanish, and *ayin ha'ra* in Hebrew, persists today in many Mediterranean, Latin American, and Middle Eastern countries.

But ancient Egyptians and other cultures also believed in the positive, protective, and healing power of the eyes. The Eye of Horus, which first appeared more than 5,000 years ago, is one of the oldest enduring positive representations of the eye, symbolizing both protection and power. The left eye symbolized the moon, and the right—known as the Eye of Ra (or Re)—represented the sun.

Whether or not we believe in the evil eye, we attribute tremendous meaning to the eyes. Indeed, eyes are usually the first thing we focus on when meeting a new person or greeting an old friend. They are the most recognizable part of the human face, if not the whole body, which is why eye masks have been used for centuries to hide the wearer's identity. Masks still play a prominent role in such festivals as Halloween and Mardi Gras, where they're used symbolically to hide the identity of their wearers from devils and other evildoers . . . or just fellow revelers.

Considered the "windows to the soul" or the "mirrors of the soul," our eyes convey the full gamut of human emotions—love, hate, happiness, anger, envy, lust, sorrow, and pain. You can laugh as well as cry through your eyes. If we know what to look for, they can also tell us—and others—much about our state of health, providing early warning signs of many diseases. No wonder doctors always look into our eyes during a physical exam.

SIGNIFICANT FACT

The American Psychiatric Association's *Diagnostic and Statistical Manual of Mental Disorders* lists the evil eye ("*mal de ojo*") as a culture-bound syndrome that affects children in Mediterranean and Latin American countries. Among its symptoms are diarrhea, vomiting, insomnia, and fits of unprovoked crying.

SIGN OF THE TIMES

The Eye of Horus is the inspiration for the "all-knowing eye" that today sits atop the pyramid on the back of the U.S. one-dollar bill. And the right eye (the Eye of Ra) is believed to be the origin of the *Rx* symbol still used today for medical prescriptions.

EYE SIGNS OTHERS CAN SEE

CIRCLES UNDER THE EYES

When we see people who have circles under their eyes, we're likely to assume the circles are due to lack of sleep—or possibly a hangover. But that's not always the case. Many of us are plagued with these unsightly signs even when we get our eight hours.

Indeed, dark circles may be something most of us can legitimately blame on our parents.

SPEAKING OF SIGNS

The face is the mirror of the mind, and the eyes without speaking confess the secrets of the heart.
—St. Jerome, 4th–5th century Greek
biblical scholar, *Letter 54*

We're all thin-skinned underneath our eyes, but some of us inherit thinner, paler, and more transparent skin than others. The thinner, lighter, and more transparent the skin, the greater the likelihood of our having bluish-tinged blood vessels around our eyes. Other factors may also come into play. For example, dark circles can be a telltale sign of a woman's hormonal status. Many women become paler during menstruation or pregnancy, causing the blood vessels under their eyes to become more visible. And some medications—such as aspirin, Coumadin (warfarin), and other blood thinners—can dilate the blood vessels underneath the eyes, making blood vessels and circles more evident.

Circles under the eyes can also signal some underlying medical conditions, the most common of which are *eczema* (a skin condition characterized by dry and itchy skin) and allergies. In fact, dark circles are often called "allergic shiners." Allergies cause blood veins to become congested and blood to pool under the eyes. To make matters worse, people with allergies often have itchy eyes. When they rub their eyes, they can injure and bruise the delicate tissue beneath them, causing further darkening.

Dark circles can also be a red flag that you've been doing too much sunbathing. We all know that excess sun exposure causes the skin to redden or darken; the skin around our eyes is no exception.

BAGS UNDER THE EYES

The puffy pouches of skin under the eyes that we call bags can be signs of depression, as can circles. But it's more likely the insomnia and crying that often accompany depression—rather than the depression itself—that are to blame. Crying can cause fluid retention, and the fluid tends to pool under the eyes. Menstruation, pregnancy, excess salt intake, and certain medications, such as antidepressants and birth control pills, can also cause fluid retention and, of course, bags. Conversely, bags can also be a sign of the dehydration caused by alcohol, so they may be our body's way of telling us that we're drinking too much. Fluid can also accumulate around our eyes while we sleep, which is why we often wake up with puffy eyes.

STOP SIGN

Sleeping with your head elevated may help reduce fluid retention under the eyes. And many people find that applying cold cucumber slices or chilled tea bags over their eyes for 5 to 10 minutes helps reduce bags and puffiness.

Bags under the eyes are also a common warning sign of *hypothyroidism,* an underactive thyroid. (See Appendix I.) Droopy eyes (see **Droopy Eyelids,** below), feeling cold all the time, and having dry skin and hair are other classic signs.

SIGNIFICANT FACT

The skin of our eyelids is the thinnest skin on our bodies.

Lastly, both bags and dark circles are major—and unavoidable—signs of aging. As we age, the skin under our eyes becomes thinner and loses its elasticity, causing it to sag and form pouches. The bags themselves cast dark shadows, making the circles appear even darker.

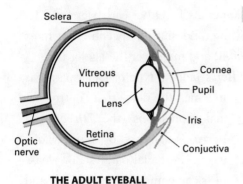

Sclera

Vitreous
humor

Lens

Retina

Optic
nerve

Cornea

Pupil

Iris

Conjuctiva

THE ADULT EYEBALL

CREASES UNDER THE EYES

Ever look at a family photo album and notice a common facial trait—a crease or prominent skin fold in the lower eyelid? If so, it can be a sign of a genetic condition called the *Denny-Morgan skin fold,* which is actually an eye sign of *eczema.* In addition to eczema, people with Denny-Morgan skin folds—and many of their relatives—often suffer from *hay fever* or *asthma.*

DROOPY EYELIDS

While "bedroom eyes" may be sexy, droopy eyelids—medically known as *ptosis*—can be a real turn-off. Unfortunately, they're usually just another unavoidable sign of aging. As we grow older, the tendon-like tissue on top of the eyes tends to stretch and our eyelids droop. Age-related ptosis typically affects both eyes and is usually nothing to worry about. However, the lids may droop so low they can block a person's vision.

Sometimes droopy eyelids are not age-related but a sign of *hypothyroidism* (see **Bags Under the Eyes**, above) or *myasthenia gravis (MG),* an autoimmune disorder that causes muscle weakness in various parts of the body, especially the eyes. (See Appendix I.) Other early signs of MG are double vision, difficulty swallowing, and slurred speech. It is most common in women under the age of 40 and men over the age of 60.

Ptosis can also be a marker for *Bell's palsy,* a type of facial paralysis in which the nerve that controls facial expressions (the *7th cranial nerve*) is damaged by injury or disease. The facial paralysis or weakness can come on quite quickly and usually affects only one side of the face. Other common eye signs of Bell's palsy are having difficulty closing your eyes or blinking, which in turn can result in excess tearing or dry eye. (See **Watery Eyes** and **Dry Eyes,** below.) The good news is that the paralysis from Bell's palsy is rarely permanent; it usually resolves without treatment in 2 to 3 weeks. Only about 10% of sufferers experience a recurrence—often on the opposite side of the face.

SIGN OF THE TIMES

The droopy-eyed dwarf Sleepy, one of the Seven Dwarfs in Disney's 1937 film *Snow White and the Seven Dwarfs,* was reportedly modeled after a friend of Walt Disney's who had myasthenia gravis.

A single droopy eyelid can be part of a cluster of nerve-damage-related signs that, taken together, are known as *Horner's syndrome.* Typically, Horner's affects just one side of the face. The eye on the damaged side will have a constricted (small) pupil, an eyeball that recedes into the face, and an iris that changes color. (See **Eye Color Changes,** below.) Interestingly, that side of the face doesn't sweat (*anhidrosis*). Horner's usually signals a serious injury to the facial nerves, possibly from a head or neck injury, a spinal cord disorder, a brain tumor, or even lung cancer. In rare cases, Horner's is present at birth.

DANGER SIGN

If your previously normal eyelid suddenly droops, call your doctor immediately or go to the emergency room. You may have a brain injury or tumor. If your drooping eye is accompanied by double vision, weakness in your facial muscles or other parts of your body, severe headache, or difficulty speaking or swallowing, you may be having a stroke.

Having one droopy eyelid may also be an early warning sign of a number of serious neurological or systemic disorders, some of which can be life-threatening. For example, a droopy eyelid on one side of the face may be an early warning sign of a *stroke, infection, tumor, diabetes,* or *brain aneurysm* (a thin, weakened area in a blood vessel wall that may rupture).

BULGING EYES

We've all seen people whose eyes seem to pop out at us. Remember Rodney Dangerfield? And who can forget the bug-eyed Igor, played by Marty Feldman, in Mel Brooks's film *Young Frankenstein*?

When prominent eyes are present since birth, they're usually a benign family trait. But if your eyes start to bulge later on—a condition called *exophthalmos* (sometimes spelled *exophthalmus*) or *proptosis*—it can be a serious sign of *hyperthyroidism,* an overactive thyroid. (See Appendix I.) Both Dangerfield's and Feldman's bulging eyes were the result of this condition. In fact, bulging eyes are one of the most common signs of *Graves' disease,* the leading form of hyperthyroidism. (See Chapter 6.)

Graves' disease is an autoimmune disease in which antibodies attack the thyroid gland, causing it to produce an excess amount of thyroid hormone and a person's metabolism to speed up, sometimes to dangerous levels.

The excess hormones also can cause muscles, tissue, and fat in and around the eyes to swell and push the eye forward, resulting in bulging eyes, known as *Graves' ophthalmopathy* or *thyroid eye disease.* About

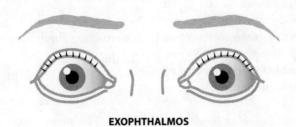

EXOPHTHALMOS

half the people with Graves' disease also have thyroid eye disease. In fact, in some people, the eye signs are apparent before the other common signs of Graves' disease, which include palpitations, hand tremors, insomnia, heat intolerance, and excessive hunger, thirst, and weight loss. Graves' disease is about eight times more common in women than men, and women are five times more likely to have thyroid-related exophthalmos than men.

WARNING SIGNS

Signs of Graves' ophthalmopathy are:
- Bulging eyes (*exophthalmos*)
- Puffy eyelids
- Gritty eyes
- Excessive tearing
- Double vision
- Blurred vision
- Decreased vision
- Jittery back-and-forth eye movements (*nystagmus*)

If you're not sure if your eyes or someone else's are bulging or just prominent, look closely at the whites of the eyes (*sclera*). In most people, including those with prominent eyes, you *cannot* see the whites showing between the tops of the irises and the upper eyelids. However, in people with exophthalmos, the whites of the eyes above or below the irises are very noticeable. People with thyroid eye disease also have difficulty blinking, making them look like they're staring.

Eyes that don't blink enough may not produce enough tears, causing them to feel dry, gritty, and irritated. In some cases, completely closing the eyes becomes difficult, making them vulnerable to serious in-

SIGN OF THE TIMES

President George H. W. Bush was diagnosed with Graves' disease eighteen months after his wife, Barbara, was found to have the disorder. The chances of Graves' occurring so soon in 2 unrelated people living in the same household—a phenomenon known as *conjugal Graves' disease*—is about 1 in 3 million. To this day, some conspiracy theorists think that the water in the White House, Camp David, or the Bushes' Kennebunkport home was poisoned by none other than Saddam Hussein!

jury, including *corneal ulceration* (an open sore on the cornea) and possibly perforation. Finally, if the eyes can't fully close at night, sleeping becomes extremely difficult.

WARNING SIGN

Exophthalmos usually affects both eyes. If it suddenly occurs in only one, it can be the sign of a hemorrhage or serious inflammation in the eye socket (orbit) or sinus passage.

If your bulging eyes are not caused by thyroid disease, they may be a sign of an *infection* or *glaucoma,* or something even more serious, such as *leukemia* or an *eye tumor.* Treating the underlying thyroid or other condition often will help the eyes recede back to normal. But sometimes people are left with permanently bulging eyes. In very severe cases of exophthalmos, surgery may be needed to decompress the eyeball.

INSIDE-OUT EYELIDS

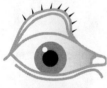

**FLOPPY EYE
SYNDROME**

If you roll over one night and your partner's upper eyelid is turned inside out, don't freak out. The everted eyelid is most likely the result of a recently identified condition, *floppy eyelid syndrome,* which is most often seen in obese men. Floppy eyelids can be a sign of several serious obesity-related problems, including *sleep apnea, hypertension,* and *diabetes.*

GROWTHS ON THE EYELID

While not as bizarre-looking as inside-out eyelids, growths on the eyelid—like growths anywhere on the body—are unwelcome and worrisome intruders. And they can be disturbing to both you and your vision. If the growths are yellowish, they're probably *xanthelasmas,* painless—albeit ugly—fatty deposits under the skin. They're usually found on the inner corner of the upper eyelid. (When found on other parts of the body, they're called *xanthomas.*) Regardless of where they're located, they tend to occur in people over age sixty, and women are about twice as likely as men to have them.

WARNING SIGN

If you have yellow growths on your eyelids as well as yellow skin (*jaundice*) and intense itching (*pruritus*), these can be signs of *primary biliary cirrhosis* (*PBC*), a rare but potentially deadly liver disease. About 90% of PBC sufferers are middle-aged women. It's a progressive autoimmune disease that leads to cirrhosis, liver failure, and death.

Although xanthelasmas themselves are usually harmless, half the time they're markers of high levels of LDL cholesterol (the bad cholesterol) or low levels of HDL cholesterol (the good cholesterol), both of which are risk factors for heart disease. And because xanthelasmas can grow quite large, there's a chance they can interfere with eyesight and may need to be removed surgically. They may, however, grow back.

LUMPS AND BUMPS ON THE EYEBALL

If you notice a white or yellowish lump or bump on the white of the eye, don't panic. This creepy-looking blob is probably nothing more than the sign of a benign and fairly common eye condition with the unpronounceable name *pinguecula*. They tend to appear off to the side of the eyeball nearest the nose. (When they extend to the surface of the cornea, they're called *pterygia*.) Pingueculae are actually age spots, and like age spots on the skin, they result from cumulative sun exposure. These slow-growing eyeball bumps are also a telltale sign of overexposure to wind and dust. But unlike many other sun-related age spots, they usually don't become cancerous. They may, however, become irritated and grow so large they interfere with eyesight or make contact lenses hard to fit.

STOP SIGN

Even if *pingueculae* and *pterygia* are removed surgically, they tend to grow back bigger and more quickly than before. Wearing sunglasses with 100 percent ultraviolet ray protection may help prevent or delay their return.

BLOODSHOT EYES

When you see people with bloodshot eyes, you may think that they've been crying or had one too many. And you may be right. When you "cry your eyes out," the small blood vessels in the eyes dilate or become inflamed. Drinking too much alcohol can have a similar effect.

Bloodshot eyes can also signal that you're suffering from a cold or allergies. But if your bloodshot eyes last for several days and you're taking an anticoagulant medication (blood thinner), you may be having an unfortunate reaction. These drugs can sometimes cause hemorrhages in the eye as well as other parts of the body.

WARNING SIGN

If your eye is more pink than red, feels irritated, and has a watery discharge, you probably have *conjunctivitis*, a highly contagious eye infection. Without taking special precautions, chances are it will spread to your other eye—as well as to others in your household.

Chronic bloodshot eyes can be a red flag that you have *ocular rosacea. Rosacea* is a common skin condition that causes the face to become red, oily, and pimply. (See Chapter 9.) About 60% of people with rosacea also have ocular rosacea, which can cause other eye problems such as watery eyes, dry eyes, eye irritation, and light sensitivity. If left untreated, ocular rosacea can lead to corneal damage and impaired vision.

DANGER SIGN

Seek medical attention immediately if you have bloodshot eyes along with any of the following signs: severe headache, blurred vision, mental confusion, nausea and vomiting, or seeing halos around lights. You may be having an attack of *acute glaucoma* (a sudden increase in eye pressure), which, without prompt treatment, can lead to blindness.

YELLOW EYES

Having red eyes is one thing, but when the whites of our eyes turn yellow, it may conjure up images of aliens or the devil. Yellow eyes are a hallmark of *jaundice,* a condition in which the skin and eyes turn yellow from too much bilirubin, an orange-yellow pigment in the blood. Jaundiced eyes are often warning signs of serious liver disease, such as hepatitis, cirrhosis, or liver cancer. Yellow eyes can also signal pancreatic cancer, sickle cell anemia, and yellow fever, a tropical disease transmitted by a mosquito bite.

Yellow eyes may signal *Gilbert's syndrome,* a hereditary form of jaundice, which affects up to 10% of Caucasians and does not usually cause medical problems. Indeed, other than high bilirubin levels, people with this syndrome have no other signs or symptoms and have a normal life expectancy. The jaundice is often mild and sometimes occurs as a result of stress, infection, fasting, or exertion.

SPEAKING OF SIGNS

When a man speaks the truth in the spirit of truth, his eye is as clear as the heavens. When he has base ends, and speaks falsely, the eye is muddy, and sometimes asquint.

—Ralph Waldo Emerson,
Spiritual Laws, *Essay IV*

SPOTS ON THE EYES

Have you ever gazed into someone's eyes and noticed the whites of their eyes have spots on them? Bright red spots that look like blood on the sclera can be a sign of a painless and usually benign condition called *subconjunctival hemorrhage.* These spots are actually blood vessels that burst from forceful coughing, sneezing, vomiting, or an eye injury. They can be a sign of high blood pressure, especially in older people.

Red spots on the eye can also be a sign of *focal senile translucency of the sclera,* a condition in which calcium deposits cause dark areas to appear on the white of the eye. Although disconcerting, this condition is yet another normal, harmless, but unappealing sign of aging. Recurring red spots, however, can signal high blood pressure or a blood-clotting disorder.

RINGS AROUND THE IRIS

If you see a ring, an arc, or a halo circling a person's iris, you may have spotted another common eye sign of aging, *arcus senilis*. Also known as *corneal arcus,* these yellowish white rings are composed of cholesterol that deposits around the iris or the rim of the cornea. They're more common in men than in women and in people of African descent than in whites. Fortunately, they don't impair vision. There is some controversy surrounding the medical significance of these rings. They've been linked to xanthelasmas (see

SIGNIFICANT FACT

The cornea is the only living tissue in the body that does not contain blood vessels.

Growths on the Eyelid, above), as well as high cholesterol levels, diabetes, high blood pressure, and other conditions that raise the risk of heart disease and stroke. Young people with corneal arcus rings are at particular risk. A recent Danish study showed that women with arcus senilis were more likely to have a shorter life span than women without this sign.

DIFFERENT-SIZED PUPILS

One in five people has one pupil that's smaller than the other, a condition known as *anisocoria*. While most people with this sign are born that way, some develop it later in life.

The size of the pupils (the dark openings in the center of the eye through which light travels to the retina) is determined by the iris, which opens and closes to regulate the amount of light entering the eye. Pupils reach their peak size during our teen years and start shrinking until we're about 60. After that, they remain pretty much the same size.

Having different-sized pupils is usually a normal inherited trait that generally doesn't cause any problems. But the pupil of one eye can change size as a result of physical trauma, or it can happen for no apparent reason (*idiopathic*). When such changes occur, they often revert back to normal on their own.

SIGN OF THE TIMES

When he was 12 years old, rock star David Bowie got into a fight over a girl and his rival punched him in the eye. The result: two different-sized pupils.

Sometimes, however, a sudden change in the size of one pupil can signal a life-threatening condition such as a cerebral hemorrhage, brain tumor, meningitis, encephalitis, or aneurysm.

DANGER SIGNS

Seek immediate medical attention if you notice that you have two different-sized pupils in any of the following situations:
- After an eye or head injury
- Accompanied by a headache, nausea, vomiting, blurred vision, or double vision
- Accompanied by fever, light sensitivity, stiff neck, or headache that worsens when you bend forward
- Accompanied by severe eye pain and/or loss of vision

EYE COLOR

Like the color of our hair, the color of our eyes is determined by our genes. Most people have black or brown eyes. By comparison, blue eyes are relatively rare and most often found in people of northern European descent. Finland has the highest concentration of people with blue eyes—fully 90% of its population.

SIGNIFICANT FACT

People with blue eyes tend to have larger pupils than those with brown eyes.

Green eyes are even rarer; they tend to be found among people of Celtic,

Germanic, and Slavic descent, with Hungary taking the lead. And green eyes are so common among the Pashtuns that these Afghans and Pakistanis are called *hare ankheim vaale*—"the green-eyed people."

WARNING SIGN

Blue-eyed people are more likely than dark-eyed people to suffer eye damage from the sun. As a result, they tend to be at greater risk of developing cataracts and macular degeneration, a progressive eye disease that is one of the leading causes of blindness. No matter what the color of your eyes, wearing dark glasses can help protect eyes from these and other eye disorders.

Eye Color Changes

Just as our genes program the color of our eyes, they appear to play a role in age-related eye-color changes. About 10 to 15% of Caucasians experience eye color changes during adolescence or adulthood. The eyes of hazel- or brown-eyed children may become lighter, while those of gray- or green-eyed children tend to darken. And many blue-eyed people notice that their eyes become brighter blue as they get older, giving them a china-doll-like appearance.

Mismatched Eye Color

If you meet someone whose eyes are two different colors, you may think he or she put in a mismatched pair of colored contact lenses by mistake or is trying to look trendy. But it's more likely *heterochromia iridium,* a condition in which a person has two different-colored eyes—or irises, to be precise. Although fairly common among dogs, cats, and horses, heterochromia iridium is quite rare in humans. In another form of this condition, *heterochromia iridis,* the different colors are in the same eye, creating a piebald or

SIGN OF THE TIMES

The ancient Greeks feared people with blue eyes, believing they could cast the evil eye. To ward off the threat, they carried around blue charms that looked like blue eyes. Today, many Greeks—as well as other southern Europeans and Middle Easterners—still carry these blue amulets.

mottled effect. Either type of heterochromia can be congenital or acquired by disease, injury, or drug reaction.

Eyes of different colors can be another of the cluster of signs known as *Horner's syndrome.* (See **Droopy Eyelids,** above.) Mismatched eye color can also be a sign of *Fuchs' heterochromic iridocyclitis*, an eye disorder that tends to strike young adults. Often people with this condition—which typically affects only one eye—also have floaters and blurry vision and are at increased risk of developing cataracts or glaucoma.

SIGN OF THE TIMES

Aristotle, Alexander the Great, and Louis Pasteur were reported to have two different-colored eyes. Some modern-day celebrities—including Kate Bosworth, Jane Seymour, Kiefer Sutherland, and Christopher Walken—do as well.

Having mismatched eye color can also signal a type of glaucoma called *pigmentary glaucoma,* which primarily affects young men. Other signs of pigmentary glaucoma may include blurry vision and occasional pain after physical exercise or exertion.

WARNING SIGN

Interestingly, some eye drops used to treat glaucoma, such as latanoprost (Xalatan), can darken the iris. If you put the drops in only one eye, they may leave you with two different-colored eyes. Doctors may not prescribe this to blue-eyed people because the darkening of the eyes is permanent. Eyelids and eyelashes have also been seen to darken.

Two different-colored eyes can also be a tip-off that you've had an eye injury. And it can be a rare sign of both nonmalignant skin tumors and skin cancer.

TEARS

We all know that tears are a normal sign of intense emotions, both sadness and joy. But few realize that tears can be of both the emotional and the lubricating varieties and that the two kinds have a different biochemical composition. Scientists have recently discovered that emotional tears actually contain more protein and certain stress-related hormones than the tears that normally bathe the eyes.

Tears are made up of three layers: a layer of sticky mucus (helps the tears adhere to the eye and protects the cornea), a watery layer (moistens and nourishes the eye), and an oily layer (seals the tears on the eye and helps slow down their evaporation).

Our tears continuously bathe and cleanse our eyes, flushing out dust and debris that can damage our sensitive corneas. Our tears can even kill the bacteria that enter our eyes. And with each blink, our lids spread lubricating, cleansing tears over the entire surface of the eye.

SIGN OF THE TIMES

Copious tears have not always been a shameful sign of weakness. In the 8th century, the most famous medieval French warrior, Roland (Charlemagne's nephew, who was memorialized in the epic poem the *Song of Roland*), died in battle. When his fellow knights—more than 20,000 strong—learned of his death, they were so overcome with grief that they wept openly and with such intensity that they fainted and fell from their mounts.

Watery Eyes

If tears continuously cascade down your face, it may not be anything to cry over, but it's nothing to laugh about, either. Just as a runny nose can be a sign of allergies, so can runny eyes. So if you frequently find yourself overflowing with tears but not overwhelmed with sadness or happiness, it may mean that your environment is just too windy, dusty, or flower-filled for you.

Occasionally, too many tears can signal *vitamin B$_2$ (riboflavin) deficiency.* This vitamin is essential for the health of your eyes and skin. Watery eyes can also be a sign of *rosacea,* the skin condition that can cause your eyes and skin to turn red. (See **Bloodshot Eyes,** above, and Chapter 9.) Or they can signal more serious conditions such as a blocked tear duct, a nasal polyp, or Graves' disease. (See **Bulging Eyes,** above.)

Dry Eyes

When our eyes don't produce enough tears or our tears contain chemicals that cause them to evaporate too fast, we wind up with *dry eye,* which usually affects both eyes. People with dry eye often complain of eyes that feel sandy or scratchy. This condition is very common, particularly as we age, and is more so in women. A woman's body naturally produces less oil as she ages, especially after menopause because of reduced estrogen production. With less oil, the tear film can't seal in the watery layer, so tears evaporate too quickly.

SIGNIFICANT FACT

On average, a blink lasts one-third of a second, and we blink about 15 times a minute. That's about one blink every four seconds.

Ironically, watery eyes may actually be a sign of dry eye. If tears aren't sticky enough to stay in place and moisten your eyes, out they spill. And chronic dry eye, like watery eyes, can be a sign that you're not living in the best environment for you. Indeed, people who live in hot, dry, windy places, at high altitudes, or in overheated or excessively air-conditioned homes are at increased risk of having dry eye.

Dry eye is a common reaction to certain prescription or over-the-counter medicines such as antihistamines, antidepressants, and antihypertensives. It may also be your body's way of telling you that you're reading too much or putting in too many hours at your computer. The more we concentrate and stare, the less we blink and the less often our eyes are lubricated.

While dry eye is usually not a particularly serious sign, it can be a sign of Graves' or other thyroid disease, as can watery eyes. (See **Bulging Eyes,** above.) Dry eye can also signal some other serious autoimmune disorders, such as rheumatoid arthritis and *systemic lupus erythematosus* (**SLE** or lupus), a very serious, chronic disorder characterized by inflammation of and damage to many parts of the body. (See Appendix I.)

If you have dry eye, dry mouth, and joint inflammation, that combination of signs points directly to another serious autoimmune disorder: *Sjögren's syndrome.* (See Appendix I.) In this disorder, the body attacks its moisture-producing glands. Women are its prime victims. Indeed, fully 90% of Sjögren's sufferers are women, and the average age of onset is the late 40s. If untreated, Sjögren's can severely damage the cornea and adversely affect other organs, especially the mouth, digestive tract, and female reproductive system.

If you have dry eyes that treatment doesn't help, blink a lot, have other uncontrollable facial spasms, and have trouble keeping your eyes open even when you're not tired or bored, you may have the telltale signs of a rare neurological disease called *Meige's syndrome.* If your chin thrusts forward when you blink, it's a sure-fire sign of Meige's, also known as *hemifacial spasm* and *Brueghel's syndrome.*

Meige's syndrome, which tends to strike people in middle age, affects more women than men. People with this treatable syndrome are unfortunately often misdiagnosed as having a psychological disorder. In most cases, Meige's is more annoying and embarrassing than debilitating. But in severe cases, the spasms may cause the mouth to clamp shut, making eating and talking extremely difficult. And in rare cases, it can signal a brain tumor.

SIGN OF THE TIMES

Meige's syndrome was named after Henry Meige, a French neurologist who first described this condition in 1910. But this condition was known hundreds of years before. Indeed, in his painting *De Caper,* the famous Flemish artist Brueghel (1525–1569) depicted a woman whose face and neck were contorted by this condition. The term *Brueghel's syndrome* is also used—along with *Meige's syndrome*—to describe this condition.

EYE TWITCHES

Have you ever sat on a bus and had your eye start twitching uncontrollably? You may be afraid that your fellow passengers think you're winking at them. Not to worry. While you might feel and fear the twitching, it's probably not very noticeable to others. What you're most likely having is *lid myokymia,* a harmless, but annoying and distracting, involuntary spasm of the eyelid.

Eye twitches—which can affect either the upper or lower eyelid—are usually nothing to be concerned about. Fatigue, stress, or too much caffeine can set them off,

SIGN OF THE TIMES

In some cultures, blinking was yet another way to inflict the evil eye on someone. And the term *blinker* was used in parts of the British countryside to describe those who possessed the evil eye. Even sick cows were said to be "blinked," because it was thought the evil eye had been cast upon them.

as can staring at a computer screen, television, or any other flickering light. The twitches may last for only a few seconds, may occur for several days at a time, or may come and go.

While usually benign, lid myokymia can be an early sign of Meige's syndrome (see **Dry Eye,** above) or *blepharospasm,* with which it's often confused. With blepharospasm, however, the eyelids repeatedly shut tight, rather than twitch. The eyes are also often irritated and very light-sensitive. And unlike myokymia, untreated blepharospasm can lead to severe vision impairment.

STOP SIGN

Quinine (in the form of tonic water—with or without the gin) has long been used to stop eye twitches. If you don't like the taste, gently pressing the twitching spot may help, at least temporarily. In most cases, the twitching stops after a good night's sleep or when you become less stressed. (Interestingly, tonic water can also help relieve nighttime leg and foot cramps.)

DARTING EYES

If you see someone with shifty eyes, he may be up to no good. Or his shifty eyes may be a sign of *nystagmus,* a condition that involves jerky, involuntary eye movements that usually occur in both eyes. Nystagmus can cause one or both eyes to move back and forth, up and down, or even around in circles. The eye movement may be constant or episodic and last for a few minutes to several hours. Unless it affects their vision or others mention it, people with nystagmus may be unaware of having this condition.

Nystagmus can be a sign of Graves' disease (see **Bulging Eyes,** above), as well as a sign of inner ear disorders such as *Ménière's disease* (see Chapter 3). And it can also sometimes signal more serious conditions such as a stroke or brain tumor.

EYE SIGNS ONLY *YOU* CAN SEE

FLOATERS

Have you ever seen spots or flecks floating in front of your eyes? You may think you have dirt or something worse in them, but you can't feel it. If you try to rub the spots away, they remain or get worse. That's because what you're noticing is not dust or debris. Rather, what you're most likely seeing are "floaters"—medically known as *opacifications* or *condensations*.

Floaters can look like flecks, cobwebs, hairs, dust particles, or tiny insects gliding across your field of vision. But they're not actually *on* the eye's surface, which is why they don't disappear when you rub your eyes. Rather, they're tiny clumps of *vitreous humor* (also spelled "humour"), a jelly-like fluid inside the eyeball. You're most likely to notice floaters when you look directly at a solid light-colored background, such as a white wall or clear blue sky. They usually last for only a few seconds or possibly minutes, and they come and go with changes in head position. Although usually permanent, many people stop noticing them after a while.

If floaters bug you, you're not alone; virtually everyone sees them from time to time. People who are very nearsighted and those who have had eye surgery are more likely than others to see floaters. Floaters usually first appear when we're teenagers and tend to increase in frequency as we get older. This is because the vitreous humor starts to pull away from the retina as we age. Small shreds of the gel then break off and float across our field of vision.

Floaters are usually just an annoying sign of aging. They can, however, sometimes signal a serious problem, especially if: you start seeing a lot more than usual, you see larger ones, you notice them when looking at dark as well as light backgrounds, or they cluster in one spot. These are all common early warning signs of cataracts, eye inflammation, eye hemorrhages, or other serious eye problems. And a sudden shower of floaters may signify something even more dangerous, such as a retinal tear or detachment. A retinal detachment is a medical emergency requiring immediate attention—undiagnosed and untreated, it can lead to permanent blindness.

DANGER SIGN

If you have a sudden change in vision—especially if you start seeing double or things start to look blurry—call your doctor right away or head to the emergency room. If you've had a recent injury to your head or face, it may be a sign of a concussion. If not, it still may signal a serious condition that requires immediate medical attention.

FLASHES

If you've ever hit or been struck on your head, you probably saw stars or flashes of light—medically known as *phosphenes.* Phosphenes can be seen when your eyes are either open or closed, often appear in the peripheral vision, and last for just a few seconds. Some people say these flashes look like shooting stars; others describe them as "a shower of sparkles."

The sensation of seeing flashing lights is called *photopsia.* Students, writers, and others who keep late or long hours sometimes experience photopsia when they're sleep-deprived or after pulling all-nighters. In addition to a whack on the head, sneezing or vigorously rubbing your eyes can set off a shower of these flashes.

DANGER SIGN

An increase in flashes—or flashes along with floaters—can be a sign of a retinal tear, a retinal detachment, or an acute vitreous detachment, all of which require immediate medical attention. Even when these conditions are treated, the flashes may persist for several months.

Occasional flashes are normal and usually no cause for concern. Most flashes, like floaters (see **Floaters,** above), are a normal sign of aging. But persistent or frequent light flashes can be a sign of low blood pressure, especially if they occur after you stand up quickly. Light flashes can also be a harbinger of migraine headaches; in fact, they're the most common visual sign—called an *aura*—of an impending migraine. Spasms of blood vessels in the brain cause these flashes.

WARNING SIGN

Recently the famous Nurses' Health Study found that women who suffer from migraines that are preceded by a visual aura are at increased risk of heart attack or stroke. Researchers don't yet know if the same is true for men.

Paradoxically, some migraine sufferers have a visual aura but not a headache. (Migraines don't always involve head pain.) In addition to eye flashes, this type of migraine—sometimes called *ophthalmic migraine* (aka *silent migraine*)—can cause other visual disturbances, as well as nausea and nasal congestion. Some people with eye migraines do go on to have migraine headaches years later.

PHANTOM VISIONS

Seeing floaters and flashes is one thing, but what if you start seeing fanciful flowers, flocks of flying birds, or frolicking ferrets that aren't really there? Don't freak out—you're probably not going crazy. You're most likely experiencing the classic signs of *Charles Bonnet syndrome*. In this condition, mentally healthy people see phantom visions, a form of visual hallucinations. Some have reported seeing such pleasant visions as groups of children, animals, vivid visual patterns, or even bucolic country scenes. They can last a few seconds or minutes, and they may recur periodically over months or even years.

SIGN OF THE TIMES

Charles Bonnet syndrome was named for the 18th-century Swiss naturalist who was the first person to describe this condition. His nearly blind 87-year-old grandfather had been seeing people, birds, carriages, buildings, and patterns that weren't there. Apparently Bonnet himself experienced similar phantom visions as his own eyesight deteriorated.

Some people claim they not only enjoy these visions but can change them at will. Others, however, find them embarrassing and frightening, fearing they may be losing their mind. But Charles Bonnet syndrome sufferers—unlike many psychotic individuals—are aware their visions are not real. And their visions are *never* accompanied by auditory hallucinations, a common sign of psychosis.

The famous 19th-century English poet Alfred Lord Tennyson was said to have suffered from failing eyesight, floaters, and phantom visions. "These animals... are very distressing and mine increase weekly; in fact, I almost look forward with certainty to being blind," he purportedly wrote to his aunt about his phantom visions.

Rather than losing their mind, people with phantom visions are likely to be losing their eyesight. Indeed, in most cases, phantom visions are signs of poor or deteriorating eyesight or other eye problems, such as glaucoma, cataracts, and especially *age-related macular degeneration* (*AMD*). AMD is a very common and serious degenerative eye disease that is the leading cause of vision loss in adults. Women, whites, people with light-colored eyes, smokers, and the obese are at increased risk. AMD also appears to run in families.

The following are signs of age-related macular degeneration:
- Blurry vision
- Poor night vision
- Straight lines appear wavy or bent
- Poor central vision or blank spots in center of the visual field
- Difficulty recognizing faces
- Difficulty adjusting to low light conditions
- Increased difficulty seeing at a distance
- Difficulty distinguishing colors or colors are less vivid
- Increased difficulty doing detailed activities, such as sewing or reading
- Phantom visions

Phantom visions are actually fairly common among people with poor eyesight; estimates run from 10 to 40%. They're thought to be similar to *phantom limbs*—the experience of feeling an arm or leg after an amputation—and may be the failing eyes' attempt to compensate for lost vision by recalling past images. Simply improving home lighting may help make the visions disappear. Interestingly, when some people with deteriorating eyesight become totally blind they no longer "see" the phantom visions.

When phantom visions occur in people with normal eyesight, it can signal Alzheimer's disease, Parkinson's disease, stroke, or another neurological condition. Unfortunately, people who experience phantom visions are often hesitant to tell their doctors because of fear of being labeled psychotic, demented, or drug-addicted. As a result, they may not get the treatment needed to help save their eyesight or treat the underlying cause.

WARNING SIGN

If you notice that you're having difficulty seeing things to the side of you or you are losing your peripheral vision, it may be a forewarning of glaucoma, degeneration of the retina, or even a stroke.

LIGHT SENSITIVITY

The sun makes us all squint—a phenomenon medically known as *photophobia,* which literally means "fear of light." But if you notice you're shielding your eyes or reaching for your sunglasses more often than before and you're also sensitive to indoor lights, your photophobia may be signaling any number of conditions. Light sensitivity is more common in blue-eyed people and migraine sufferers than others.

SIGN OF THE TIMES

The first cataract surgery was performed in the 5th century B.C. by Sushruta, the father of Indian surgery and ophthalmology.

Photophobia can signal such eye disorders as cataracts, retinal detachment, and corneal abrasions. It can be a reaction to such drugs as tetracycline, doxycycline, belladonna, and even quinine, or it may be a sign of a vitamin B_2 deficiency. Light sensitivity can also be a dead giveaway that a person has been abusing alcohol, cocaine, amphetamines, or other drugs.

Sometimes photophobia signals some serious but treatable conditions—such as measles, hypertension, and Graves' disease (see **Bulging Eyes,** above)—as well as such potentially life-threatening diseases as meningitis, encephalitis, botulism, rabies, and mercury poisoning. However, you'd have other, much more serious signs in addition to light sensitivity if you suffered from any of these potentially deadly disorders.

NIGHT BLINDNESS

Night blindness can gradually creep up on us, making it increasingly difficult to see what lurks in the dark, creepy or otherwise. Not seeing well in the dark—medically known as *nyctalopia*—is yet another normal, annoying sign of aging.

Night blindness is also a common sign of a cataract. And it's one of the earliest warning signs of vitamin A (retinol) deficiency, which can lead to very dry corneas and retinal damage.

SIGN OF THE TIMES

In ancient Egypt, eating liver was thought to cure night blindness. Thousands of years later, it was discovered that liver is rich in vitamin A. Researchers today have found that vitamin A slows the progression of retinitis pigmentosa.

However, if you're young and have night blindness, it may be the first sign of a genetic condition called *retinitis pigmentosa*, a degenerative disease of the retina that may lead to severely impaired vision in some cases.

COLOR-VISION CHANGES

Among "acid freaks" and others who use hallucinogens, seeing things morph into weird colors is a fairly common, not to mention much sought-after, experience. But if you're not into drugs, seeing abnormally colored objects—medically known as *chromatopsia*—can be an early warning sign of diabetic eye disease. Even slight fluctuations in blood sugar levels can very quickly produce these vision changes. If you do have diabetes, these color vision distortions can make it very difficult for you to monitor your blood sugar levels using color-coded urine test strips. So this is yet another reason to say no to cake.

WARNING SIGN

It's not unusual for athletes with diabetes to experience vivid color vision changes after strenuous practice sessions or games. This can be a very early warning sign of diabetic eye disease.

If things start looking yellow, however, you could have a type of chromatopsia called *xanthopsia*. Xanthopsia can be a warning sign that you have jaundice from a serious liver disease. If you're seeing yellow and/or halos around objects and are taking digitalis (a drug commonly used to treat certain kinds of heart disease), it may be a red flag that you have *digitalis toxicity*. This is a medical emergency; it can lead to heart failure, cardiac arrhythmias, and death.

SIGN OF THE TIMES

It's believed that Van Gogh's extensive use of the color yellow in such paintings as *Starry Night* and *Sunflowers* was the result of the digitalis he took for mania and epilepsy. Digitalis—which is derived from the fox-glove plant—has been used for centuries to treat anxiety, mania, convulsions, and heart disease.

If your male partner, who's always seen life through rose-colored glasses, starts complaining that things are looking blue, it may not be because he's depressed. Rather, it may be a sign that he's taking too much of a good thing. Indeed, seeing a blue tinge on objects—often accompanied by light sensitivity—is one of the most common side effects of Viagra, Cialis, and Levitra, which are used to treat erectile dysfunction (ED).

WARNING SIGN

If you've been taking drugs to treat erectile dysfunction and suddenly can't see out of one or both eyes, stop taking the drug and call your doctor right away. This may be a sign of *non-arteritic ischemic optic neuropathy (NAION)*, a condition that can lead to blindness. Men with retinal or other eye diseases should avoid these products altogether.

SIGNING OFF

The eye signs described may or may not require medical attention. If you have any doubts, see an ophthalmologist as soon as possible. But if you have any eye signs that involve pain, sudden changes in vision (especially with nausea or vomiting), or persistent flashes of light, see your doctor immediately.

And, of course, whether or not you have eye signs, keeping up with regular eye exams not only can help preserve your vision but also may help detect the earliest signs of many other types of medical problems. Regular eye examinations are particularly important if you have diabetes. The following are eye specialists who diagnose and/or treat eye and vision problems:

- *Ophthalmologist:* A medical doctor who specializes in diagnosing and treating eye diseases and disorders.
- *Optometrist:* Although not a physician, a doctor of optometry (OD) has specialized training in vision problems and in treating vision conditions with glasses, contact lenses, low-vision aids, and vision therapy. Optometrists can test for such conditions as glaucoma, cataracts, and macular degeneration and prescribe medications for certain eye diseases.
- *Optician:* Also not a physician, an optician specializes in making and adjusting eyeglasses and other optical aids from prescriptions written by an ophthalmologist or optometrist.

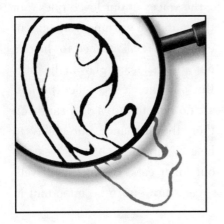

CHAPTER 3

LISTENING TO YOUR EARS

Do your ears hang low?
Do they wobble to and fro?
Can you tie them in a knot?
Can you tie them in a bow?

—POPULAR CHILDREN'S SONG

It's not only children who find ears silly. Most of us don't take our ears—at least our outer ears—very seriously. Without a doubt, they're two of the more ridiculous-looking parts of our faces. And deformed or unattractive ears have been the objects of surgical correction for thousands of years. On the flip side, the importance of our ears has been recognized for at least as long as we've been trying to beautify them. Indeed, they've played a prominent role in mythology and religion. The ancient Egyptians, for example, considered the ear a receptacle of life's breath. They believed that the "air of life" entered the right ear, while the "air of death" entered the left. And the Egyptians, like people in many other ancient cultures, pierced their ears, believing that metal kept evil spirits from invading the body. Centuries later, sailors pierced their ears thinking it would improve their eyesight.

The ear was also a significant symbol in early Christianity; Mary was said to have conceived Jesus through her ears by "hearing the word of God." In fact, many early Christian paintings portrayed the Baby Jesus descending from heaven toward Mary's ear.

It's no wonder that ears have attained such symbolic significance; for without hearing, there's neither music, the voices of our loved ones, nor the sounds of warning from our enemies. We're all attuned to the role our internal ears play in hearing. But our outer ears, called *pinnas*, are nothing to turn a deaf ear to, either; they enhance our ability to hear by funneling sound waves into our inner ears. Beyond their well-known ability to process sound waves, ears turn out to be important in sending signals about our health.

SIGN OF THE TIMES

The oldest mummified human in the world has pierced ears. Discovered in an Austrian glacier in 1991, this 5,000-year-old mummy has holes in its ears measuring about ¼ to ½ inch in diameter.

EAR SIGNS OTHERS MAY NOTICE

RED EARS

When we see someone with bright red ears, we might assume they're embarrassed about something, and we may be right. Whenever we blush, our ears—as well as our faces and other visible body parts—often turn crimson. But red ears can also be a warning sign that it's time to get out of the sun. Because our ears tend to stick out from our bodies, they're on the front lines for sunburn.

SIGN OF THE TIMES

The first case of plastic surgery on the ear was described in 600 B.C. by the Indian surgeon Sushruta. He used flesh from a patient's cheek to fashion a missing earlobe.

Red ears may be red flags for ear infections as well as such skin diseases as *psoriasis* or *rosacea*. (See Chapter 9.) They can also signal a condition, aptly named *red ear syndrome,* in which one ear typically becomes red, hot, and sometimes painful. Various seemingly innocuous triggers—such as touching your ear, turning your neck, chewing, sneezing, or

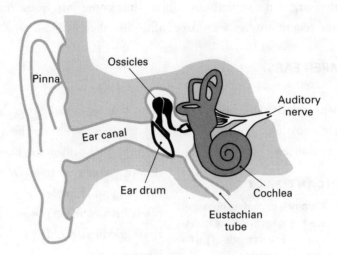

EAR ANATOMY

coughing—can set off red ear syndrome, which primarily affects children and young adults. But regardless of age, it's often associated with migraine headaches that affect the same side as the red ear.

EARLOBE CREASE

SIGN OF THE TIMES

Statues of the Roman emperor Hadrian (A.D. 76–138) clearly show that he had ear creases on both ears. Historians note that he also had frequent nosebleeds, a common sign of hypertension. His death was likely due, they believe, to heart failure brought on by the high blood pressure.

If you look in the mirror and see a diagonal crease on your earlobe, it may be a sign that you've slept too long on that ear or you've been talking on the phone too long. But if the crease is always there, it may be a sign that you're at increased risk for coronary heart disease (CHD) or diabetes. Such creases appear to run in families, and they tend to be more common in men than women.

Since first reported in the literature in 1973 by S. T. Frank, the connection between heart disease and diabetes and the *diagonal ear crease—*

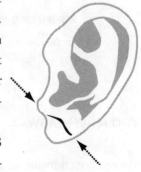

EARLOBE CREASE

or *Frank sign,* as it's sometimes called—has come into question. However, some recent studies seem to confirm his observations.

MISSHAPEN EARS

People with misshapen ears are often born that way. And while they may be merely a cosmetic concern, deformed ears can sometimes be a sign of an inherited disease or congenital (present at birth) disorder. These conditions, which include Down syndrome and Fragile X syndrome, often involve more obvious and serious medical problems than misshapen ears.

SIGNIFICANT FACT

Mammals (including humans) are the only living creatures with outer ears made of cartilage rather than simply skin.

An oddly shaped ear can be an acquired sign as opposed to a congenital sign, as in the case of the notorious *cauliflower ear.* This is usually a tip-off that the ear has been punched or injured repeatedly, which is why the condition earned the title *boxer's ear.* However, cauliflower ears don't appear only in people who play contact sports. Anyone who's had a serious blow to the ear can wind up with this

SIGNIFICANT FACT

Your ears (and your nose) grow throughout your life.

unsightly sign. Sharp blows to the ears cause blood clots to form around or even in the ear cartilage. If not treated immediately, scar tissue builds up and the ear becomes permanently deformed.

WARNING SIGN

Cauliflower ear in nonathletes can be a telltale sign of spousal or other physical abuse.

TOO MUCH EARWAX

We're all well aware of earwax—that annoying, sticky, sometimes smelly stuff that can seep out of our ears. Medically known as *cerumen,* earwax is mainly composed of cerumen (a type of wax) and sebum (a type of oil), to say nothing of more than 40 other substances including dead skin cells. There are actually two types of earwax—wet and dry—and the type we have is genetically determined.

If you sometimes find earwax on your pillow, it's most likely a healthy sign that your ear is self-cleaning. Earwax protects our ears from water, fungus, and a host of germs. It also traps dust and dirt that routinely enter our ears—or even the occasional stray fly, ant, or other tiny unwanted creature. But if your ear is turning out gobs of wax, it may be a weird warning sign that you're on a diet that's too low in fat.

SIGNIFICANT FACT

People of European and African descent usually have wet, sticky, brown earwax; those of Native American and Asian descent tend to have dry, brittle, gray, or beige earwax. Women with wet earwax appear to be at increased risk for breast cancer. Indeed, Japanese women with European-like wet earwax have a higher rate of breast cancer than Japanese women with Asian-type dry earwax.

Excess earwax can also be a telltale sign that you're overzealously cleaning out your ears. Ironically, aggressive cleaning can cause your ear to become impacted with wax. And putting an inflexible object in your ear, such as a cotton swab or even your pinky, can perforate your eardrum and introduce dangerous bacteria, fungi, and viruses.

STOP SIGN

If you hear that ear candling—medically called *ear coning*—is a good way to remove earwax, listen up. Several recent studies have snuffed out this theory. They've shown that ear candling, which involves placing a hollow, wax-coated tube in the ear and lighting the far end, can not only damage your inner ear but burn your ear and face as well. One study found the practice made the problem worse—melted candle wax was actually deposited in the ear.

WATERY EAR DISCHARGE

We're all pretty used to our noses running, but when wet stuff leaks out of our ears, it's another matter. As with earwax, watery discharge from the ear—medically known as *otorrhea*—can be a clue that the ear is cleaning itself.

But ear drainage may signal several conditions that if left untreated can progress to more serious problems. For example, a painless drainage from the ear can be a sign of a respiratory tract infection or a bacterial, fungal, or viral infection in the ear.

DANGER SIGN

 If you have blood-tinged ear discharge, call your doctor immediately or go to the emergency room. It can be a sign of a tumor in the external or middle ear canal. If you've recently had a blow to your head or head surgery, you may have spinal fluid leakage, which can be life-threatening.

And if you have yellow, pus-like discharge, which may or may not be smelly, it can point to a permanently perforated eardrum or to a chronic middle ear infection—medically known as *chronic otitis media*. Chronic middle ear infections can cause hearing loss, ear polyps, *cholesteatomas* (skin-like cysts in the middle ear), and *mastoiditis* (a serious infection of the bony structure behind the ear). If untreated, both cholesteatomas and mastoiditis may lead to meningitis and even death.

SIGN OF THE TIMES

 Oscar Wilde suffered from ear infections all his life. After his release from prison, he finally had surgery on his ear—apparently to remove cholesteatomas. Unfortunately, he died a few weeks later of meningitis. Ironically, his father, Sir William Wilde—a leading eye and ear specialist—pioneered a surgical procedure to treat mastoiditis and remove cholesteatomas, which was probably used on his son. This procedure is known to this day as Wilde's incision.

EAR SIGNS ONLY WE SENSE

ITCHY EARS

Having an itch where you can't scratch—like in your ear—can drive you crazy. Not surprisingly, itchy ears are another sign of allergies or skin conditions such as eczema and psoriasis. Itchy ears can also be a sign that you're cleaning your ears too much, leaving them dry and unprotected from lurking bacteria and fungi. (See **Too Much Earwax,** above.) In fact, itchy ears may mean that you don't produce enough earwax in the first place.

An ear itch can also be an early sign of *swimmer's ear (otitis externa)*, a condition in which the external ear canal is infected with bacteria or fungi. Later signs of swimmer's ear often include yellowish, sometimes foul-smelling, discharge and pain. While swimmer's ear may sound innocuous, if untreated, it can progress to an extremely painful and potentially life-threatening condition called *malignant otitis externa,* a bone infection.

SIGN OF THE TIMES

Ancient Egyptians used borax, duck grease, and cow's milk to treat middle-ear infections. Human milk was Hippocrates's drug of choice. He also advised his patients to drink sweet wine and avoid the sun, wind, and smoke-filled rooms.

STUFFY EARS

Do you sometimes feel that your ears are stuffed with cotton? If you've ever flown, you're probably no stranger to the feeling of fullness in the ear. Indeed, this sign is known as "airplane ear" or *barotrauma,* and it is caused by a rapid change in pressure (usually the result of changes in altitude). It's common among pilots, scuba divers, mountain climbers, and roller coaster enthusiasts.

The same sensation may mean that the ear is literally stuffed—with excess wax, bits of cotton swab, or even an unwelcome insect. On a more serious note, it

SIGN OF THE TIMES

Our ear patterns, like our fingerprints, are unique. Almost a century before fingerprints were used, Johann Caspar Lavater (1741–1801), a Swiss theologian and physiognomist, classified and identified people by their outer ear patterns. Since then, earology or otomorphology (the study of the shape of the outer ear) has been used periodically by forensic scientists to identify criminals. "Ear prints" are also still occasionally—albeit unsuccessfully—introduced as evidence in U.S. courts.

can signal several medical conditions, including middle ear infection, temporomandibular joint disorder (TMJ), and cholesteatomas. (See **Watery**

Ear Discharge, above.) Clogged ears can also be a sign of *Ménière's disease,* an inner ear disorder that can cause periodic bouts of dizziness, hearing loss, and ringing in the ears. It can also signal *otosclerosis,* a degenerative disease that affects bone in the middle ear. (See **Gradual Hearing Loss,** below.)

RINGING IN YOUR EARS

Do you hear music and there's no one there? If so, you may be experiencing a sign of *tinnitus,* a condition in which you "hear" ringing or other sounds that aren't really there. Indeed, the word *tinnitus* comes from the Latin meaning "to tinkle or to ring like a bell." Some tinnitus sufferers hear pulsating sounds, whooshing, roaring, and even crickets chirping. Some hear these sounds in one ear, others in both. These sounds can range from mildly annoying to maddening.

> ### SIGN OF THE TIMES
>
>
> In the 19th century, physiognomists believed that ear size and shape could predict criminal behavior. Cesare Lombroso (1835–1909), the leading Italian criminologist of his day, wrote that "ears of unusual size, or occasionally very small, or standing out from the head as do those of the chimpanzee" were signs of a born criminal.

They can interfere with everything you do, from working and watching TV to sleeping, driving, and even having sex.

Depending on its underlying cause, tinnitus may be temporary, but for most people it's a lifelong problem. Many of us will experience tinnitus at some point in our lives. For some, it may be another one of those irritating signs of aging. In fact, in elderly people tinnitus and hearing loss often occur together.

> ### STOP SIGN
>
>
> Tricking your brain to get its mind off the ringing sound sometimes helps mask tinnitus. If, for example, you're trying to sleep and your tinnitus is coming in loud and clear, play low music or keep a softly ticking clock by your bedside. Concentration and relaxation exercises sometimes help, too.

If your taste in music runs toward heavy metal rather than easy listening, ringing in your ears can be a sign of ear nerve damage from excessively loud music.

Like the feeling of fullness in your ears (see **Stuffy Ears,** above), a ringing sound can be a sign of excessive earwax or an indication that a foreign object—such as a cotton swab or even an insect—has taken up residence in your ear. Occasionally, a ringing sound in your ears can be a reaction to something you've eaten or drunk, such as alcohol and caffeine, or a medicine, especially aspirin and other nonsteroidal anti-inflammatory drugs (NSAIDs) and some antibiotics.

SIGN OF THE TIMES

Medieval artists earmarked earwax as a useful binding material for paints. When mixed with pigments, the concoction was used to paint illuminated manuscripts.

Tinnitus can also signal an ear or sinus infection, TMJ, otosclerosis, or Ménière's disease. (See **Stuffy Ears,** above.) This sign can also sound a warning bell for a myriad of non-ear-related maladies, including allergies, anemia, hypothyroidism, hypertension, hardening of the arteries (*arteriosclerosis*), and even a head injury. Rarely, tinnitus is a danger sign of a brain tumor or a brain *aneurysm*—a weakening in a blood vessel wall that can lead to a stroke.

WARNING SIGNS

If you have recurrent bouts of the signs below, you may have Ménière's disease.

- Hearing loss
- Dizziness or vertigo
- Ringing in the ears
- Feeling pressure or fullness in the ear

HEARING YOUR HEARTBEAT

If you occasionally hear what sounds like your heart beating, you may be right. Many of us notice this sign when we lie down in bed with our ear on the pillow. In this case, it's a normal, albeit annoying, sign that can interfere with your hearing and sleep, not to mention your peace of mind. But some people experience a similar sensation, described as a throbbing sound only in one ear, even when they aren't lying down. Called *pulsatile tinnitus* (aka *objective tinnitus,* because the sound is audible during a physical examination), it can be a warning sign of a vascular disorder, such as a heart murmur, hypertension, or hardening of the blood vessels in your heart or neck.

SPEAKING OF SIGNS

Nature has given man one tongue, but two ears, that we may hear twice as much as we speak.

Zeno of Elea, *Fragments VI,* 5th century B.C.

DANGER SIGN

If you hear a throbbing sound or heartbeat in one ear and have a severe headache, call your doctor or go to the emergency room. You may be experiencing signs of an impending stroke.

SENSITIVITY TO SOUND

Do you find the sound of your mother-in-law's voice not just annoying but unbearably loud? It may not be her fault, especially if other voices and everyday noises hurt your ears. You may, in fact, have the classic sign of extreme sound sensitivity, medically known as *hyperacusis,* a rare condition affecting about one in 50,000 people. Extreme sound sensitivity is sometimes a harbinger of tinnitus. (See **Ringing in Your Ears,** above.) Ironically, people with impaired hearing sometimes become supersensitive to certain sounds.

SIGN OF THE TIMES

Beethoven not only started losing his hearing when he was 27 (apparently from otosclerosis) but also suffered from hypersensitivity to noise and tinnitus. By the time he was 50, he was totally deaf. Yet he continued to compose until his death a few years later.

Noise sensitivity can be a reaction to the artificial sweetener aspartame as well as some antibiotics, analgesics, and allergy medicines. It can also signal *magnesium deficiency.* And finding normal noises annoying can be a sign of head injuries and whiplash, as well as depression and *post-traumatic stress syndrome*. It can also be a clue to a number of medical disorders such as chronic ear infections, certain autoimmune disorders, Lyme disease, TMJ, or Bell's palsy, a type of facial paralysis.

HEARING A LOUD EXPLOSION WHEN SLEEPING

If you're awakened by sounds that go "BOOM!" in the night and no one else hears them, it may in fact be all in your head. Being periodically awakened by hearing a loud explosion in your head is a sign of a bona fide, albeit rare, condition aptly called *exploding head syndrome*. People with exploding head syndrome are awakened by an oftentimes terrifying, brief loud noise when falling asleep or shortly thereafter. Doctors don't know why some people—

SIGN OF THE TIMES

Students sometimes complain of hypersensitivity to sound during exam week. They may not be malingering and avoiding studying. Their sound sensitivity may be the result of drinking too many aspartame-containing diet sodas.

usually older adults—experience this bizarre hearing problem. Luckily, you don't need to duck under the covers for long, since these explosions tend to stop after a few weeks or months. So while this may be one of the scariest-sounding signs you'll hear about, it's probably one of the most benign. The good news is, it's not linked to any medical problem.

HEARING SOUNDS THAT OTHERS DON'T

If you start hearing things such as songs that aren't playing, it can be pretty scary. Certainly, we've all heard how schizophrenics often hear voices, called *auditory hallucinations*. But hearing sounds that others don't can also be a sign of some other serious disorders, such as *Lewy body dementia (LBD)* or *Parkinson's disease dementia*. It's unclear whether

SIGNIFICANT FACT

The smallest bone in your body is in your ear. Called the *stirrup,* this bone is about the size of a grain of rice.

these neurodegenerative disorders or another neurological problem is responsible for the auditory hallucinations or whether it's the drugs used to treat them.

GRADUAL HEARING LOSS

Do you find yourself saying "What?" all the time? Or does your family complain you keep the TV on too loud? For most people, hearing loss silently creeps up on them. In older people, this type of hearing loss—medically known as *presbycusis*—is quite common, occurring in 75% of people over the age of 60, and affects more men than women. The hearing loss may progress so slowly that you don't realize it until you're using your eyes to read other people's lips more than you're using your ears to listen to them speak.

SPEAKING OF SIGNS

What a humiliation for me when someone standing next to me heard a flute in the distance and I heard nothing, or someone standing next to me heard a shepherd singing and again I heard nothing. Such incidents drove me almost to despair; a little more of that and I would have ended my life—it was only my art that held me back.

—Ludwig Van Beethoven, excerpt from a letter to his brothers, 1802

People with presbycusis usually have impaired hearing in both ears and have difficulty hearing high-pitched sounds. Fortunately, presbycusis seldom ends in total deafness.

SIGNIFICANT FACTS

Men are forever being accused of not listening to the women in their lives. Now there's scientific basis for this charge. According to a government survey, men do indeed have poorer hearing than women. The researchers also found that black adults had keener hearing than white adults.

Hearing loss isn't just an "old folks' disorder." Gradual hearing loss does occur in young people and can be a sign of *otosclerosis*. (See **Stuffy Ears**, above.) Indeed, this ear condition—which can begin in the teens—is the leading cause of hearing loss in young adults.

Young white middle-class women are at highest risk for otosclerosis, and hormonal changes during pregnancy may worsen the condition. While otosclerosis usually occurs in both ears, sometimes it affects only one, especially in men. The exact cause of otosclerosis is unclear, although it's thought to be a hereditary condition.

Gradual hearing loss may also be sounding an alarm that you've been working or playing in very noisy places. In fact, frequenting loud restaurants or working in a typical factory—both of which have decibel levels around 85—is enough to ruin your hearing over time. By comparison, the decibel level of a jet engine hovers at 140 and a rock concert can reach 150.

SIGN OF THE TIMES

In the 1960s and '70s, it was loud rock concerts. In the new millennium, it's MP3 players that doctors say are the latest culprits in what is feared will become an epidemic of hearing loss.

In addition, slowly progressing hearing loss may be a wake-up call that any number of medical conditions may be brewing, including hypothyroidism, rheumatoid arthritis, diabetes, and kidney disease. Hearing loss in one ear—particularly if you have ringing in the ears and dizziness—may be a sign of *acoustic neuroma,* a tumor on the nerve that controls hearing; it is noncancerous but can be life-threatening.

SUDDEN HEARING LOSS

If you wake up one morning to find that you suddenly can barely hear the birds chirping outside your window or your kids fighting over their breakfast cereal, you may be experiencing *sudden sensorineural hearing loss (SSNHL),* more commonly called *sudden deafness.* SSNHL is defined as a hearing loss in one ear that develops over 72 hours or less. In fact, one in three people with SSNHL wake up deaf in one ear. For the other SSNHL sufferers, the first sign of hearing loss is often

SIGN OF THE TIMES

HEAR—Hearing Education and Awareness for Rockers—was started by a group of famous rock musicians who lost some of the ability to hear after years of playing and listening to loud music. They wanted to call attention to the dangers of overly loud music and give tips on how to protect the ears and hearing.

a popping sound or a ringing in the ears. (See **Ringing in Your Ears,** above.)

This type of hearing loss is most common in people between the ages of 30 and 60 and is often accompanied by dizziness. Hearing returns in one-third of cases and slightly improves in another third. Unfortunately, one-third of people who experience SSNHL remain deaf in that ear.

Sudden hearing loss may be a sign of several serious ear conditions, including Ménière's disease (see **Stuffy Ears,** above) and acoustic neuroma (see **Gradual Hearing Loss,** above). It may also signal *autoimmune inner ear disease (AIED)*, an inflammatory ear condition in which the body's immune system goes amok and mistakenly attacks the cells in the inner ear. Often people with this condition will have other signs besides hearing loss, such as light-headedness, lack of coordination, tinnitus, or a feeling of fullness in the ear.

Sudden hearing loss may also point to such serious systemic disorders as multiple sclerosis, sickle cell anemia, bacterial or viral infection, lupus erythematosus, and cancer.

WARNING SIGN

Here are two more reasons to quit smoking: smokers are 70% more likely to suffer hearing loss than nonsmokers, and living with a smoker doubles your risk of hearing loss.

SIGNING OFF

Ear signs are sometimes so subtle that we barely notice them, while others come in loud and clear. Remember, any sudden hearing loss, pain, unusual discharge, or bleeding from the ear requires an immediate call to your doctor or trip to the emergency room.

Other ear and hearing signs can be evaluated and treated by various health care professionals. In general, a physical examination by a primary care clinician—such as an internist, general practitioner, family physician, nurse practitioner, or physician assistant—should include a peek into your ears and a periodic hearing test as you age.

Because our ears are so interrelated with our other sensory organs, many ear specialists are also trained in diagnosing and treating nose and throat disorders. Here are some medical doctors and hearing specialists whom you may need to call to check your ears.

- *Otolaryngologist* (also known as *otorhinolaryngologist*): A medical doctor who specializes in diagnosing and treating ear, nose, and throat diseases and disorders.
- *Otologist*: An otolaryngologist (see above) with additional training in ear disorders.
- *Audiologist*: A health care professional trained in testing for and treating hearing and other ear-related problems such as poor balance. They can also fit hearing aids and perform other hearing rehabilitation services.

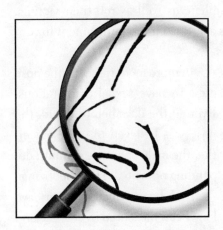

CHAPTER 4

YOUR NOSE
KNOWS

'Tis enormous!...Know
That I am proud possessing
  such appendice.
'Tis well known, a big nose is
  indicative
Of a soul affable, and kind,
  and courteous,
Liberal, brave...

—EDMOND ROSTAND,
"CYRANO DE BERGERAC," 1897

The nose has loomed large throughout human history. In virtually every age and culture, people have tried to please and appease their gods, saints, and even demons by burning fragrant incense. The nose had a prominent role in the Bible: according to the book of Genesis, God created humankind by blowing the "soul of life" into Adam's nostrils. Later, Jacob asked God to send humans a sign so they would know when they were fatally ill, giving them enough time to repent before dying. Jacob's wish was granted: God created the sneeze. No wonder ancient Israelites believed sneezing portended a medical disaster. On the other hand, Aristotle and his fellow ancient Greeks believed a sneeze was a good omen.

No strangers to aesthetics, ancient cultures knew the value of a good-looking nose. In fact, the first recorded nose jobs were described on papyrus by Egyptian physicians around 3000 B.C. By 600 B.C., Sushruta, the Indian surgeon, had perfected the technique, which was much needed, because countless noses were being cut off at the time by vicious gangs of bandits who wanted to humiliate as well as rob their victims. Hacking off noses (and genitalia) was also a common punishment for unfaithful spouses in those good ol' days.

SIGN OF THE TIMES

During the 19th and early 20th centuries, swollen noses were thought to be a sign of sexual obsession and habitual masturbation. Some doctors performed nasal surgery—on both men and women—to stop what they considered abnormal sexual practices and thoughts. Even Freud prescribed such surgery for some of his female patients. Ironically, scientists have since discovered that the nose, much like the penis and the clitoris, swells during sexual excitement.

In more modern times, the nose grew to have sexual connotations. Even in the days before Freud, the nose was believed to represent either the male or female genitals, depending on who did the theorizing.

Both beauty and character have long been measured by the size and shape of one's nose. In the 18th and 19th centuries, for example, pseudoscientists known as physiognomists characterized people's moral makeup and personalities by their noses, ears, and other visible body parts.

In 1848, George Jabet, an English physiognomist, went even further. In his book *Nasology, or Hints Towards a Classification of Noses,* he wrote that the nose was actually shaped by the mind. He classified noses into six categories, each with its own aesthetic and moral attributes. It's now widely believed that Jabet—who penned his book under the name of a woman (Eden Warnick)—wrote it as a joke.

SIGN OF THE TIMES

Unfortunately, Jabet's nose theories—as well as those of other physiognomists—were taken seriously and helped pave the way for racism in Nazi Germany and elsewhere.

Our noses play a key role not only in how the world perceives us but also in how we perceive the world. After all, it's our noses that let us smell the roses. And because smelling and tasting are so intricately connected, our noses help us savor the taste of our favorite foods and drinks.

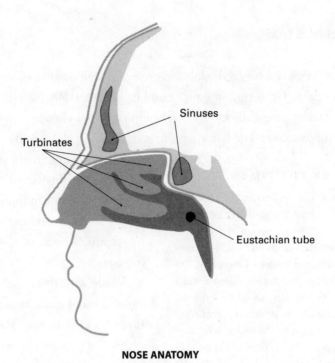

NOSE ANATOMY

But our noses can also smell trouble. Indeed, what our noses smell or don't smell—as well as what comes out of them—can tell us what problems may be brewing inside our bodies. And yes, even how they look can give us hints about our health.

NOSE SIGNS OTHERS MAY NOTICE

A RED NOSE

While kids may associate red noses with clowns and Santa's reindeer Rudolph, most adults realize they're common signs of sunburn, allergies, and colds. But a red nose can be a red flag for *rosacea*, a condition in which the skin becomes abnormally reddened. (See Chapter 9.) And sometimes it's a telltale sign of alcohol abuse. Alcohol causes the blood vessels near the skin surface to dilate, giving the skin a reddish hue.

A BULBOUS NOSE

Most of us view a big, red, globular nose as a sign of alcoholism, and we may be right. However, an equal number of teetotalers have this condition, which is medically known as *rhinophyma* but is commonly referred to as *bulbous nose*. The late comedic actor W. C. Fields could be a poster boy for this condition, which is seen almost exclusively in men over 40 years of age. A bulbous nose is actually a severe—though relatively rare—form of rosacea. (See **A Red Nose**, above.)

People with this condition usually have other nasal signs, such as excess or thickened nose skin. Because of the increased number of oil glands in the nose, another sign of rhinophyma is waxy, greasy, yellow skin.

SIGN OF THE TIMES

Charles Darwin had a bulbous nose. Because of it, he almost literally missed the boat to the Galapagos Islands on his way to coming up with the theory of evolution. The captain of the ship, the HMS *Beagle*, was a disciple of the famous physiognomist Lavater. Darwin wrote in his autobiography that the captain "doubted wheather [sic] anyone with my nose could possess sufficient energy and determination for the voyage."

Although bulbous nose is medically benign, its unsightliness can cause embarrassment and social problems. Plastic surgery is an option, but the condition may return.

A CREASE OVER THE NOSE

Have you ever seen someone with a crease on the bridge of the nose? If so, it may be a sign of a serious nasal allergy. The crease is the result of what's called the *nasal salute*. Allergy sufferers—particularly those who have year-round allergies—often try to relieve their unrelentingly itchy noses by repeatedly rubbing them with the palms of their hands in an upward motion. The result: a crease or wrinkle across the bridge of the nose.

SPEAKING OF SIGNS

A gentleman with a pug nose is a contradiction in terms.

—Edgar Allan Poe

SUN SNEEZING

We all know that dust, dander, pollen, pepper, and perfume are common sneezing triggers. But the sun? If you sneeze when you go out in the sun, you're not alone. In fact, about one-quarter of us experience this sign, which is known by many names—*photic sneeze reflex, solar sneeze reflex, light sneeze reflex,* and last but not least *autosomal dominant compelling helio-ophthalmic outburst syndrome* (aka *ACHOO syndrome*). Although the exact cause of this phenomena is unknown, it may be due to a crossover of sight and smell reflex signals in the brain. Described since ancient Greece, ACHOO syndrome hasn't gotten much play in the scientific literature because it's both common and totally medically meaningless. It's usually ignored by its sufferers, too, because this nasal outburst stops as quickly as it starts.

SIGN OF THE TIMES

The Egyptians thought that looking at the sun and sneezing was good luck.

INABILITY TO SNEEZE

While sneezing—medically called *sternutation*—is actually a healthy sign that our nose is doing a good job clearing itself of nasal intruders, not being able to sneeze when you feel the urge is . . . well, nothing to sneeze at. It can signal a brain tumor. And sometimes people recovering from a stroke find it hard to sneeze. A psychiatrist in India, who dubbed this condition *asneezia,* found it fairly common in patients with schizophrenia or severe depression.

SPEAKING OF SIGNS

People around the world still bless or wish a sneezer health in various ways. Here are just a few:
- In Spanish: *salud* (to your health)
- In German: *gesundheit* (good health to you)
- In Polish: *sto lat* (one hundred years)
- In French: *à vos souhaits* (to your wishes)
- In Finnish: *terveydeski* (for your good health)
- In Hebrew: *labriut* (bless you)
- In Romanian: *noroc* (good luck)

SNORING

You may be able to turn a deaf ear to sun sneezing, but snoring is hard to ignore. Perhaps you can't get a good night's sleep because your partner sounds like he's orchestrating a symphony through his nose. Or your own nasal nocturnes drive your bedmate crazy and to the living room— or analyst's couch, or even a marriage counselor.

SIGNIFICANT FACT

Sleep apnea leads to more than a poor night's sleep. People with sleep apnea are 2 to 7 times more likely to get into a car accident. And men with sleep apnea may find that their sexual performance can take a nosedive.

For some, snoring can be a very annoying telltale sign of drinking too much, especially at bedtime. Although a bottle can be hidden from one's partner, it's harder to cover up those annoying nose noises, medically known as *stertor.* Snoring can also be a warning sign of overeating. Indeed, being overweight and snoring often go hand in hand.

SIGN OF THE TIMES

Michelangelo was left with a permanently disfigured nose after a fistfight. A fellow Florentine art student, Pietro Torigiano, was so jealous of the young artist's talent that he punched him in the nose. Michelangelo—who was already shy and reclusive—became even more withdrawn. Torigiano was banished from Florence.

But snoring can be more than a noisy nuisance or caused by a behavior that you can change; it can signal a number of medical conditions, some more serious than others. Snoring may simply be a sign of nasal congestion from a cold or allergy, or it may signal a nasal blockage from a deviated nasal septum (the structure that divides the internal nose in half) or from unusually large *turbinates* (the bony nasal structures covered by mucous membranes, which help warm and cleanse air). Snoring may point to enlarged tonsils or adenoids, a large tongue, or a long uvula (that dangly thing in the back of your throat). It might also signal that either a noncancerous or cancerous growth is blocking airflow through your nose.

Snoring can be your body's way of sounding an alarm that you have a potentially serious condition called *sleep apnea.* In sleep apnea, a person may stop breathing or the breathing can become extremely shallow. These breathing cessations can happen scores of times every hour, causing the person's oxygen level to drop dramatically, which the body interprets as a medical emergency. The heart then beats faster and the blood pressure rises steeply. To make matters worse, fluctuation in oxygen levels can cause inflammation and clog the arteries. These also put a person at risk for heart attack and stroke.

SIGNIFICANT FACT

 Almost half of normal adults occasionally snore, and 25% are habitual snorers. Men snore more than women.

Sleep apnea sometimes runs in families, and it is more common in men than women. African Americans, Pacific Islanders, and Mexican Americans are at increased risk. Interestingly, Mexican Americans *are* at greater risk than other Hispanics. Being overweight, and particularly having fat around the neck, puts a person at increased risk of sleep apnea.

WARNING SIGN

If you're a snorer and are scheduled to undergo surgery, be sure to mention it to your surgeon and anesthesiologist. Snoring is a common sign of sleep apnea. Anesthesia can be risky for patients with this condition, and special precautions should be taken.

A VERY RUNNY NOSE

Having a runny nose—medically known as *rhinitis*—is usually merely a sign of a simple cold or allergy. But a continuously drippy nose may be a telltale sign of snorting cocaine, heroin, or other drugs.

If you don't do drugs and don't have a cold or allergy but clear mucus drains continuously from your nose, it can signal a serious problem, such as a tumor.

 SPEAKING OF SIGNS

When I want any good head work done, I always choose a man, if possible with a long nose.

—Napoleon Bonaparte

If your nasal discharge is thick and discolored, it may be a warning sign of a sinus infection, especially if you have bad breath, pain, or a fever as well. Difficulty breathing and a decreased sense of smell can also signal a nasal polyp. (See **Loss of Smell,** below.) Nasal polyps are usually not cancerous, but they can interfere with breathing. And although they can be surgically removed, they frequently grow back.

SIGNIFICANT FACT

Albeit rare, excessive sneezing—medically known as *intractable paroxysmal sneezing*—has been known to result in sneezes that occur up to 2,000 times a day. This exhausting condition is thought to be psychological in origin and mainly affects young adolescent girls.

WARNING SIGN

People with nasal polyps can be allergic to aspirin and other non-steroidal anti-inflammatory drugs (NSAIDs), such as ibuprofen (Advil, Motrin) and naproxen (Aleve). Because an allergic reaction to these drugs can be life-threatening, you should avoid them unless under the close supervision of your doctor.

A DRY NOSE

A dry nose can be just as irritating as a running nose. And while it's probably nothing much to worry about, it may be a sign of *Sjögren's syndrome,* a rare but serious autoimmune disease that interferes with the production of mucus and saliva. (See Appendix I.) If left untreated, Sjögren's, which primarily affects women, can lead to eye, reproductive, and other physical problems.

Dry nose is also a fairly common sign of the use (or overuse) of some medications used to treat stuffy nose, asthma, and other nose-related conditions. These include antihistamines, nasal sprays, and bronchodilators—especially those containing the muscle relaxant atropine.

If your nose is chronically dry *and* heavily crusted, you may have a rare condition called *empty nose syndrome (ENS)*. Empty nose syndrome is found primarily in people who have undergone extensive sinus or other nasal surgery for medical or cosmetic reasons. During surgery too many turbinates (see **Snoring,** above) are mistakenly removed and the nose is literally left empty. Turbinates can also be damaged during radiation therapy or by physical trauma to the nose. Empty nose syndrome sufferers describe a frightening feeling of not being able to get enough air when they breathe. Paradoxically, they often say their noses feel both empty and blocked at the same time.

Other common signs of empty nose syndrome are shortness of breath and other breathing difficulties, a dulled sense of smell and taste, an odorous nose (see **A Smelly Nose,** below), sleep disturbance, and sleep apnea. These signs often show up many years after the surgery or damage to the turbinates.

A SMELLY NOSE

Not only can our noses smell, they can sometimes be smelly. If your nose gives off a foul odor, you might not notice it, but others certainly will.

An offensive odor emanating from your nose can signal *ozena,* a

HEALTHY SIGN

Dried nasal mucus—commonly known as *snot, boogies,* or *boogers*—may seem gross and embarrassing, not to mention difficult to get rid of…at least in public. But these nasal products are a sign that your mucous membranes are doing their job—secreting a sticky substance that helps trap and encase dirt and dust, much the same way an oyster produces pearls.

SIGNIFICANT FACTS

The first-ever survey on nose picking was conducted in Wisconsin in 1991. More than 90% of responders admitted to the habit. The most common places to pick were in offices and cars. While 22% indulged 2 to 5 times a day, 1% picked compulsively—medically known as *rhinotillexomania.*

A similar recent survey in India found the rule of thumb to be four times a day. About 8% of responders were prize pickers, probing their nasal passages more than twenty times a day. And, a whopping 17% confessed to having a nose-picking problem.

chronic disease in which the nasal structure becomes atrophied. ("Ozena" comes from the Greek word for "stench.") Ozena itself is often an early warning sign of *empty nose syndrome* (see **A Dry Nose**, above) or a more serious form of this disease called *secondary atrophic rhinitis*. (The terms are often used interchangeably.) But whatever it's called, it can ruin a person's quality of life. Embarrassed by the odor, sufferers may avoid social contact, or find that others avoid them. As a result, they may become severely depressed.

SIGN OF THE TIMES

Tagliacozzi, a celebrated 16th-century Italian surgeon, wrote the first textbook on plastic surgery. He also reconstructed noses—which often fell victim to duels—by using the skin from his patients' buttocks. Unfortunately, the Church got its nose out of joint over what Tagliacozzi was doing and excommunicated him.

NOSE SIGNS ONLY YOU NOTICE

SMELLING PROBLEMS

Our sense of smell enhances our lives in countless ways: think spring gardens, exotic perfume, cookies baking, and the nose of a good bottle of

---

WARNING SIGN

When your sense of smell goes, more is at stake than you think. You're likely to lose your sense of taste as well. Indeed, two-thirds of people who seek help for smell loss also complain about taste loss.

---

wine. And familiar smells can tweak our memories and transport us back to our childhood.

More important, however, our ability to smell is critical to survival. The sense of smell alerts us to all sorts of dangers, from noxious fumes and spoiled foods to fires. If we lose our sense of smell, we increase our risk of breathing toxic gases, getting food poisoning, or getting burned.

Loss of Smell

Is your favorite perfume or aftershave no longer as fragrant as it used to be? Depending on your age, this might be yet another one of those unfortunate signs of growing older. As our hearing, sight, and memories fade with age, so does our sense of smell.

The decreased ability to smell is medically known as *hyposmia,* while the total loss of smell is called *anosmia.* To confuse matters

SIGNIFICANT FACT

Our sense of smell is the most acute of all our senses. It's 10,000 times more sensitive than our sense of taste. Indeed, up to 90% of what we perceive as taste is actually smell.

further, when the diminished ability to smell is age-related, it's called *presbyosmia.* While our sense of smell is fully developed at birth, it's most acute from our teen years to age 60. It goes downhill from there. By our 80s, we smell only half as well as we did when we were in our 30s.

WARNING SIGN

Because the sense of smell is critical to sniff out danger, anyone who has lost this sense should have smoke and natural-gas detectors throughout the home. Carefully dating all perishable food is important as well, to avoid eating spoiled food. These safety precautions are especially critical for those living alone and the elderly.

Not surprisingly, smell loss, like a stuffy nose, is often a sign that your nasal passages are clogged from a cold, allergy, sinus infection, nasal polyp, or tumor. But it may also signal a zinc deficiency. (Zinc, in fact, is sometimes used to help restore the sense of smell.) Loss of smell from these causes tends to develop gradually and is usually temporary. Once the cause is treated, the ability to smell usually returns.

SIGNIFICANT FACT

In general, women have a keener sense of smell than men; it's most acute around ovulation.

A sudden loss of smell in people over the age of 60 often signals an upper respiratory tract infection. But sudden loss of smell is also a fairly common sign of head trauma, especially in younger people. In fact, one in ten people who has had a head injury experiences smell loss, and, unfortunately, it can be permanent.

If your sense of smell isn't as sharp as before, your nose may be warning you that you've been exposed to dangerous chemicals or environmental toxins. While smell loss from these culprits can be permanent, prompt treatment may be able to restore your ability to smell.

SIGN OF THE TIMES

Ironically, cocaine was a common treatment for nasal disorders. Freud used this "magical drug," as he called it, to relieve his own chronic nose problems. Not only did he become hooked, his nasal troubles worsened.

If you've recently had nasal surgery, a diminished sense of smell can alert you to the fact that something went awry during the procedure. It can also be a reaction to radiation therapy or chemotherapy, as well as to certain drugs such as decongestants and medications for hyperthyroidism. Speaking of drugs, smell loss—like a runny nose—can result from snorting cocaine or other illicit drugs. It can also be your body's way of warning you that you're smoking or drinking too much.

DANGER SIGN

Smoking can cause loss of sense of smell, not to mention loss of life. In addition to lung and heart disease and cancer, smokers are at increased risk of causing and being in house fires.

The loss of smell can also be the only warning sign of a type of brain tumor called *olfactory groove meningioma*. The good news is that this tumor is usually not cancerous and is treatable. The bad news is that if left alone, it can grow and affect not only your sense of smell but your vision as well. Olfactory

SIGNIFICANT FACT

People with a normal sense of smell can discern about 10,000 different odors.

groove meningioma occurs more often in women than men and usually strikes people between the ages of 40 and 70.

Smell loss can also signal a whole host of other medical disorders including diabetes, hypothyroidism, epilepsy, multiple sclerosis, lung disease, and even schizophrenia.

Finally, loss of smell can be a very early sign of the neurological disorders *Alzheimer's disease* and *Parkinson's disease.* (See Chapter 7.) Unfortunately, both of these conditions are often missed or misdiagnosed in their early stages. Smell testing is an important diagnostic tool to help differentiate these neurological disorders from other disorders.

SPEAKING OF SIGNS

The taste and the sense of smell form but one sense, of which the mouth is the laboratory and the nose the chimney.

—Brillat-Savarin, the father of modern gastronomy, in *The Physiology of Taste,* 1825

Being Supersensitive to Smell

Do you turn up or wrinkle your nose at smells no one else seems to notice? Just as the young woman in the Danish fairy tale "Princess and the Pea" was overly sensitive to touch, some people are hypersensitive to odors. Medically known as *hyperosmia,* smell sensitivity is usually a benign, albeit annoying, sign. However, if you have this condition, mildly unpleasant smells can make you nauseated. But pleasant smells come in stronger, too. For example, a person with hyperosmia can often detect the scent of a woman's perfume long after she's left a room.

SIGNIFICANT FACT

The smell of rotting flesh is, literally, the worst smell in the world, according to scent scientists. This has practical applications: the U.S. Department of Defense has tried to reproduce this smell to make a better stink bomb.

Supersensitivity to smell is often thought to be a psychosomatic condition and a sign of neurosis. But don't be so quick to run off to a shrink. It can be a sign of pregnancy. And hyperosmia can signal *Addison's disease,* a serious but rare hormonal disorder that adversely affects the mucous membranes and skin. (See Chapter 9 and Appendix I.)

Smelly Smells Only You Smell

Does your mom's apple pie smell more like pizza pie lately? Rather than blaming your mother, you may want to look to your own nose. You may have the classic sign of *dysosmia,* a distorted sense of smell. But if your local greenhouse smells more like an outhouse, it may signal *cacosmia*—a condition in which things smell putrid or fecal to you but perfectly fine to others.

SPEAKING OF SIGNS

The truth of man lies in his nose.

—Ovid, ancient Roman poet

And if you're the only one in a room who smells something, it's probably a sign of *phantosmia* or *phantom odors.* Unlike phantom visions, which often involve cute animals or beautiful scenes (see Chapter 2), phantom odors are usually far from pleasant. In fact, for the most part, they're downright disgusting. Phantosmia sufferers describe such revolting smells as rotting flesh, feces, and vomit that seem to come out of nowhere.

In some people, the phantom odors may signal schizophrenia or other psychiatric disorders. In these cases, the sufferers are likely to have visual and auditory hallucinations or other serious psychiatric signs as well.

Like hypersensitivity to smell, phantom odors, dysosmia, and cacosmia can be normal signs of pregnancy. But if you're not pregnant, they may signal epilepsy. Indeed, some people experience an odor aura just before a seizure. Interestingly, distorted or odd odors, as well as phantom odors, also can be signs of a certain type of epilepsy in which no seizures occur. They might also be harbingers of an impending migraine.

DANGER SIGN

Severe odor disorders—such as those that make food smell rotten all the time—can so disrupt quality of life that they can lead to serious depression. Indeed, a University of Nebraska Medical Center surgeon reported that almost half of his patients who suffered from smell distortions had seriously contemplated suicide.

As might be expected, all these odor disorders can signal olfactory nerve damage, which can be caused by many of the same things—including infections, head trauma, surgery, environmental toxins, and drugs—that lead to loss of smell. (See **Loss of Smell,** above.)

If the underlying condition can be treated, the smell distortions or hallucinations will probably disappear. But getting an early, accurate diagnosis is key.

SIGNING OFF

Primary care physicians—family physicians and internal medicine specialists—can diagnose and treat many nasal problems, from the common cold to allergies. But many nose problems are related to other medical conditions that require special training to evaluate and manage. Keep in mind that if you have nasal pain or excessive bleeding, you should call your doctor right away.

So, who knows the most about noses? If you have a nose-related problem and need to see a specialist, you may want to consult one of the following:

- *Otolaryngologist* (also known as *otorhinolaryngologist*): A medical doctor who specializes in evaluating and treating ear, nose, and throat problems.
- *Rhinologist:* A medical doctor who is board-certified in otolaryngology and undergoes additional training in treating nasal and sinus diseases.
- *Allergist/immunologist:* A medical doctor who is board-certified in internal medicine or pediatrics and undergoes additional training in allergy and immunology.
- *Sleep disorder specialist:* A medical or other doctor who has special training in sleep medicine and has been certified by the American Board of Sleep Medicine.

help push food around our mouths so we can better chew and swallow it, to say nothing of helping us speak.

While our mouths may provide a plethora of pleasure for us and others, they can also get us into a ton of trouble. And they can both kiss *and* tell. From the color and texture of our lips and tongue to the smell of our breath, our mouth speaks volumes about what's going on inside our bodies. It's a veritable blabber-mouth about our health. It's no coincidence that one of the first things a doctor says when examining a patient is "Open your mouth and stick out your tongue."

SIGN OF THE TIMES

The ancient Babylonians and Assyrians had several effective remedies for gum disease and mouth ulcers, including rubbing the inflamed areas with onion mixed with oil and turnip seed. Both onions and turnips, it turns out, have anti-inflammatory properties.

LIPS AND MOUTH

PUFFY LIPS

Puffed-up lips on women have been a sign of beauty and sensuality for centuries. In Victorian times, young women "practiced their *P*'s"—that is, they repeated words that began with the letter *P*—in the hope of developing a permanent set of pretty, perky, and puckered lips with which to woo suitors.

SIGN OF THE TIMES

Exchanging lost baby teeth for gifts is an old European tradition dating back to Viking days. These tiny teeth were believed to ward off witches and evil. The Tooth Fairy lives to this day. A child will tuck a lost tooth under a pillow, anxiously awaiting a coin or small gift left by the Tooth Fairy. These days, the Tooth Fairy is paying about $2 per tooth, according to a national financial magazine.

Today, unless a woman is genetically endowed with luscious lips (think Scarlett Johansson), puffy lips are more likely to be a sign of collagen injections than lip exercises (think Goldie Hawn in *The First Wives Club*). But puffy or swollen lips can also signal an allergic reaction to something you've eaten, drunk, or put on your lips to beautify them.

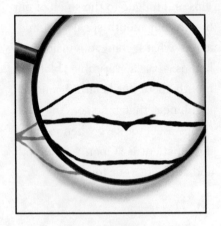

READ I
LIPS…AI
MOU

The lips, the teeth, the tip of
the tongue.
The lips, the teeth, the tip of
the tongue.

—TONGUE-TWISTING VOCAL

WARM-UP FOR ACTORS

Our lips and mouths ar
ways to some of ou
sensual pleasures: si
drinking, eating, tasting, and I
Perhaps this is why people have b
sessed with their mouths since a
times. Dating as far back as 500
remedies for mouth-related problems ranging from bad bre
toothaches have been found in the writings and inscriptions of t
cient Sumerians, Chinese, and Egyptians. Some of these conco
contained such ingredients as wine and the urine of children, b
which have subsequently been found to have antiseptic properties

Though our teeth may not have the same sex appeal as our n
and lips, they are certainly as useful. Not only do they help grind ou
but they keep our tongues from falling out of our mouths. Speak
tongues, they're not just for tasting, talking, and tantalizing. The

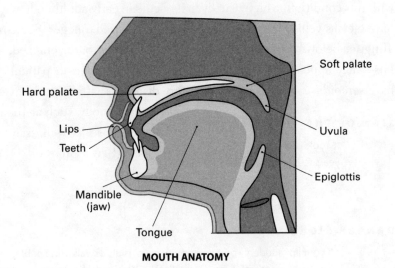

MOUTH ANATOMY

If your lower lip is puffy and has reddish or white crusty spots or sores on it, you may have *actinic cheilosis*, a progressive erosion caused by sun damage. This condition usually occurs after age 50 and is more common in men than women. Unfortunately, the damage to your lip is permanent. As with most sun-related skin problems,

SPEAKING OF SIGNS

Papa, potatoes, poultry, prunes, and prism, are all very good words for the lips, especially prunes and prism.
—Charles Dickens, *Little Dorrit,* 1855

people with fair skin are at particular risk. Actinic cheilosis is usually a precancerous condition, although it may be an early warning sign that you already have skin cancer on your lower lip.

WARNING SIGN

A bump or sore with hard edges and a brownish center on your lips may be a sign of *keratoacanthoma,* a rapidly growing skin lesion that commonly forms on the lips. Like many skin growths, it's linked to sun damage. While it may pop and go away on its own, leaving only a small depression, it may be precancerous.

Chronic puffy lips may be a sign of *Miescher-Melkersson-Rosenthal syndrome,* a neurological disorder that tends to run in families. People with this condition, which usually first occurs in early adulthood, may also have facial swelling, facial nerve palsy, and a fissured tongue. (See **Groovy Tongue,** below.) Over time, more signs—such as hard, cracked, scaly lips—may appear. These same signs are also common in patients who have *sarcoidosis,* a serious inflammatory disorder that affects many other parts of the body, such as the eyes, ears, and nose as well as internal organs. (See Chapter 9 and Appendix I.)

SIGN OF THE TIMES

It took Leonardo da Vinci 10 years to paint Mona Lisa's lips.

DANGER SIGN

If your lips suddenly puff up *and* you have trouble swallowing or breathing, seek medical help immediately. You may be having a life-threatening allergic reaction *(anaphylactic shock).*

PURSED LIPS

If you see someone with pursed lips, the word *prissy* or *mean* may be on the tip of your tongue. But pursed lips can signal a serious immunologic disorder called *scleroderma,* which causes a hardening of the skin and scarring of the internal organs. (See Chapter 9.) As the skin around the lips tightens, making it difficult to open the mouth, the lips take on a puckered, pursed look.

SIGNIFICANT FACT

Full, red lips are considered very sexy in many cultures. Scientists believe there's an evolutionary basis for this: plump lips are a visual sign of fertility. Indeed, the lips of pubescent girls swell when they're sexually excited.

DRY, CRACKED LIPS

Cold weather and chapped lips go hand in hand. While they're usually benign and caused by external factors, dry lips can be a sign of dehydration. Ironically, licking your lips can worsen the problem. Chronically dry lips can also signal a nutritional deficiency, as well as *Sjögren's syndrome,* an autoimmune disease that affects the moisture-producing glands. (See **A Dry Mouth or Excessive Thirst,** below, and Appendix I.)

BLUE LIPS

Someone with blue lips may be making a fashion statement, but it's more likely that he or she has been out in the cold too long. But blue lips may be a sign of *Raynaud's disease,* a condition in which the small arteries, usually in the fingers and toes but sometimes in other parts of the body, become constricted from the cold or emotional stress. This prevents those body parts from getting enough oxygen and turns them blue. (See Chapters 7 and 9.) Medically known as *cyanotic lips,* blue lips may also be a red flag that your body isn't getting enough oxygen because of one of several possible respiratory conditions, including pneumonia, asthma, chronic bronchitis, and pulmonary edema. Or the lack of oxygen could occur because you're a serious smoker and the carbon monoxide in the smoke is robbing your lungs and other organs of oxygen. Your blue lips could also be telling you that you're iron-deficient (anemic).

WARNING SIGN

If your lips are blue and you're pregnant, you may be iron-deficient. This is a fairly common and potentially serious problem during pregnancy.

BURNING, TINGLING LIPS OR MOUTH

Lips and mouth that tingle, burn, or even feel numb at the end of a romantic evening may be signs of a promising relationship—or they may be the earliest signs of a cold sore—medically known as *herpes simplex* (aka *oral herpes*). If so, you should kiss—or rather tell—your date goodbye for a while because herpes is highly contagious.

SIGNIFICANT FACT

Besides eating, our mouths serve another important food function: they cool or warm food to the right temperature for swallowing. This helps prevent painful "pizza mouth" and "ice cream headaches."

If you have a weird pins-and-needles feeling on your lips that isn't herpes, it may be a sign of a calcium or vitamin D deficiency. A feeling of tingliness or numbness on the lips or elsewhere—medically known as *paresthesia* (see Chapter 7)—may be one of the earliest signs of kidney disease. Oral tingling can also signal diabetes: when blood sugar isn't under control, the nerves in the mouth and other parts of the body can be damaged.

When these sensations linger, they can be signs of irritation due to broken teeth or dentures, food allergies, nutritional deficiencies, or even a reaction to your mouthwash. And a burning mouth can be a sign of *candidiasis,* a yeast infection (aka *thrush*). Thrush sometimes occurs in people who have taken antibiotics or inhaled or topical steroids, or who have dry mouth (see **A Dry Mouth or Excessive Thirst,** below). It's also common among people whose immune systems are depressed from diseases such as diabetes, AIDS, or cancer and cancer treatments. Indeed, thrush-related white patches in the mouth are often the first signs of HIV/AIDS.

STOP SIGN

 If you have burning mouth syndrome, merely switching to a different brand of toothpaste or mouthwash may help.

LIP OR MOUTH FRECKLES

Freckles may be cute on your nose, but who wants to spot them on the lips? A few oddly shaped brownish blemishes on the lips, called *melanotic macules,* are common and medically meaningless. Although no cause for alarm, these spots can stick around for years.

Freckles can also show up inside your mouth. Called *oral mucosal melanosis,* these skin-color changes are often a very early sign of *Addison's disease,* a rare hormonal disorder of the adrenal glands. (See Chapter 9 and Appendix I.) They can also signal various other hormonal conditions or changes. As with any skin blemish, if the spots or freckles change color, shape, or texture, they can be warning signs of skin cancer.

WHITE OR GRAY PATCHES IN YOUR MOUTH

Finding white or gray patches in your mouth is enough to make you lose your appetite. Medically known as *leukoplakia,* they can grow anywhere in your mouth, including on your tongue and gums. These patches, which typically appear over weeks or months, are actually excess cell growths. They can be signs of poorly fitting dentures, chewing the inside of your cheek, or other irritations. Leukoplakia can also be a reaction to mouthwash or toothpaste containing sanguinarine, an antiseptic.

If these patches show up rather suddenly, it may be a sign of thrush. (See **Burning, Tingling Lips or Mouth,** above.) But more commonly, the sudden appearance of these patches is a telltale sign of too much smoking or drinking. Unfortunately, leukoplakia in smokers and heavy drinkers is often precancerous. In fact, any color changes in the mouth of a current or past smoker can literally be a "smoke signal," an early warning of skin cancer.

WHITE STREAKS IN THE MOUTH

White streaks on the inside of the cheek, or on the gums and tongue, are usually signs of *lichen planus,* a chronic disease that typically affects the skin. (See Chapter 9.) These lesions seem to come and go at will.

Although there's some debate, lichen planus is thought in some cases to be an early sign of *hepatitis C,* a serious viral infection.

RED OR SWOLLEN GUMS

If your gums are red, rather than a healthy pink, it may be an early sign of *gingivitis,* an inflammation of the gums. Gingivitis is often a warning sign that you haven't been practicing good oral hygiene. But you're well on your way to full-blown gum disease—medically known as *periodontitis*—if your gums are swollen, soft, and tender. The bad news is that this condition, which causes the loss of the bone and connective tissues that hold your teeth in your mouth, can result in tooth loss. The good news is that with early treatment, gum disease is reversible.

HEALTHY SIGNS

 Healthy gums are pink or coral. They should also be firm and resilient when poked. And, of course, there should be no bleeding or pain.

WARNING SIGN

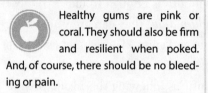 Gum disease (periodontitis) puts a person at increased risk of heart attack and stroke.

Swollen gums can be a telltale sign that you're a smoker or that you've been clenching or grinding your teeth. They can also be a reaction to certain drugs, such as oral contraceptives, antidepressants, and some heart medicines.

WARNING SIGNS

 The following are common signs of gum disease:
- Spaces between your teeth
- Pus between your teeth and gums
- Receding gums
- Bad breath
- Itchy mouth
- Mouth sores
- Changes in your bite or the way your dentures fit

Swollen gums can also signal diabetes. Indeed, one-third of people with diabetes have severe gum disease. Interestingly, treating the gum disease may help control blood sugar levels.

WARNING SIGN

Women who take fertility drugs for more than three months are at increased risk of developing gum disease. It's the estrogen in most of these drugs that can adversely affect gum tissue.

Inflamed gums can also signal the bacterial infection *Vincent's stomatitis* or *necrotizing gingivitis* (aka *trench mouth*). In severe cases they can damage oral bone and gum tissue.

A BUMP OR HOLE ON THE ROOF OF YOUR MOUTH

If you feel—or more specifically your tongue feels—a bump or lump on the roof of your mouth, don't overreact. These protrusions are most likely signs of *palatal (torus palatinus)*, bone growths on the roof of your mouth. Believe it or not, these are benign protuberances, often caused by nothing more serious than eating hard foods that irritate the palate. In fact, you may first notice these bony structures when chomping on a bagel. If these bumps get really big, as benign as they are, they can give you trouble with your speech or your dentures.

If your tongue finds a small crater in the roof of your mouth, it may be a sign of an ominous-sounding but painless and usually not serious condition called *necrotizing sialometaplasia*. These lesions are usually evidence of some injury to the inside of your mouth and sometimes heal on their own in a few months. Unfortunately some of these lesions do turn out to be cancerous.

WARNING SIGN

Recurrent *canker or mouth sores* can be an early warning sign of two serious gastrointestinal conditions, *Crohn's disease* and *ulcerative colitis*. They can also be early warning signs of the autoimmune disorder *lupus*.

A DRY MOUTH OR EXCESSIVE THIRST

Does your mouth often feel like it's made of sandpaper or stuffed with cotton? If so, you may have *xerostomia*—the medical moniker for dry mouth. Occasional dry mouth is normal and usually a sign you're dehydrated from too much salt, alcohol, or heat. It can also be your body's way of telling you that you're under stress and need to chill out.

But if you feel cool as a cucumber and your mouth is still parched, it may be a reaction to one of more than 400 prescription and over-the-counter medicines. The major culprits are antihistamines, diuretics, astringent mouthwashes, antidepressants, and some blood pressure medications.

In some cases, a parched mouth can be a dead giveaway that you're using illicit drugs such as marijuana, cocaine, and methamphetamine. Or it may be a telltale sign that you're drinking too much; alcohol is very dehydrating to the body.

SIGNIFICANT FACT

Saliva helps moisten our food so we can chew, swallow, and digest it more easily. And it washes away food and bacteria, thus preventing bad breath, tooth decay, and gum disease. Without spit, we'd lose all our teeth within 6 months!

SIGN OF THE TIMES

Realizing that anxiety can stop saliva from flowing, the ancient Chinese invented what may have been the first lie-detector test. To determine if a suspect was spitting out the truth, they put dry rice in his mouth. If the accused couldn't spit out the rice, it was considered proof positive of his guilt.

WARNING SIGN

If you put a cracker in your mouth and have difficulty chewing or swallowing it, you've flunked the "cracker test," an indicator of dry mouth.

Occasionally, dry mouth signals an injury to the salivary glands from a neck trauma, surgery, radiation treatment, or chemotherapy. Radiation-related dry mouth is permanent, while the dry mouth from chemotherapy is usually temporary.

Dry mouth may be an early warning sign of certain autoimmune disorders, including rheumatoid arthritis and *Sjögren's syndrome*. (See Appendix I.) Other common signs of Sjögren's, which primarily affects women, are dry eye, nasal dryness, and joint inflammation. Lastly, dry mouth can signal serious conditions such as Parkinson's disease, cystic fibrosis, diabetes, and even HIV/AIDS.

It's often difficult to distinguish dry mouth from excessive thirst—

SIGNIFICANT FACT

Theoretically, any substance, disease, or marker that can be detected in the blood can also be found in the saliva. To date, home and workplace saliva tests can detect illicit drugs, alcohol, HIV, hormonal changes, and even stress. Scientists have also had some success in detecting oral cancer from saliva.

one often results in the other. But extreme or unquenchable thirst can be a danger sign of advanced hyperthyroidism. (See Appendix I.) Extreme hunger is another sign. But if you're feeling hungry all the time and also have to urinate a lot, extreme thirst may signal undiagnosed or uncontrolled diabetes, which can be a precursor to a diabetic coma.

WATERY MOUTH

If your mouth spouts spit when you speak, it can be quite embarrassing. Excessive saliva may be a reaction to certain medications, especially *cholinergic drugs,* which are used to treat dry mouth and glaucoma. It's also often a sign of *gastroesophageal reflux disease (GERD)*, more commonly known as *acid reflux*. (See **Fecal Breath,** below.)

SIGNIFICANT FACT

The average person produces about a quart of saliva a day. That's about 10,000 gallons in a lifetime.

A watery mouth can signal some more serious conditions such as gastric ulcers, liver disease, pancreatitis, neurological disorders, and esophageal obstruction or cancer. On a more positive note, it may also be an early clue that you're pregnant.

THE TELLTALE TONGUE

From French kisses to the Bronx cheer, our tongues are a constant source of delight and derision.

The tongue is covered with several types of small nodules called *papillae*, some of which contain our taste buds. Like the hairs on our heads, they continuously grow and shed. The papillae on the back of the tongue shed more slowly than those in the front. They also tend to be longer, making them more susceptible to bacterial and yeast infections. Indeed, the tongue can have quite a taste for trouble.

BLACK HAIRY TONGUE

If your tongue is black but you haven't been licking a licorice lollipop or sucking a grape sourball, it may be a sign of a condition aptly named *black hairy tongue*—medically called *lingua villosa nigra*. When the tongue hairs fail to shed, they can overgrow and trap bacteria and food. As a result, the tongue turns a dark brown, green, or even dark yellow.

Black hairy tongue can be a telltale sign that you smoke, chew tobacco, and/or practice poor oral hygiene. Ironically, it can also be a sign of excessive use of mouthwash. Not surprisingly, people with this condition often have halitosis as well. (See **Bad Breath,** below.)

In addition, black hairy tongue can be a reaction to antibiotics or to stomach medications containing bismuth, such as Pepto-Bismol. It's sometimes seen in people who undergo chemotherapy or radiation treatment for head and neck cancers. Finally, black hairy tongue can also be a warning sign of poorly managed diabetes.

SIGN OF THE TIMES

Mayan and Aztec priests used tongue piercing as a way to better communicate with the gods. Today, it's a fairly common practice among youth, many of whom believe it enhances oral sex. But some who really have a taste for the exotic—and perhaps trouble—split their tongues, creating a forked tongue!

WHITE HAIRY TONGUE

Have you ever looked in the mirror and been dismayed to discover that your tongue's turned white? It may merely be from leftover toothpaste, or it might signal a reaction to peroxide-containing mouthwash. A *white hairy tongue* is, however, more often a sign of a recent fever. Or it can be a tip-off that you're a smoker or a mouth breather, or even that you're eating a diet too low in fiber.

HEALTHY SIGN

A healthy tongue should be rosy and silky soft. It should also have small, uniform bumps all over.

STOP SIGN

Gently brushing or scraping your tongue can help keep it free from bacterial and yeast infections. It can also help keep your breath smelling fresh.

BEEFY RED TONGUE

If your tongue looks more like a rare steak than ham steak and eating spicy foods makes it burn, you may have the classic signs of a condition called

bald tongue—medically known as *atrophic glossitis.* As the name implies, the tongue has lost its protective hair-like papillae, leaving it red and irritated. Like a balding head, a balding tongue tends to occur in older people. It may be a sign that their dentures don't fit well and are rubbing against their tongues. But it may also signal a vitamin B deficiency or thrush. (See **Burning, Tingling Lips or Mouth,** above.)

GROOVY TONGUE

A grooved or fissured tongue may not sound gross—that is, until you hear the medical term for it: *scrotal tongue.* Also known as *lingual tongue,*

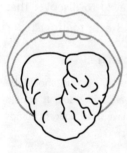

SCROTAL TONGUE

scrotal tongue is quite common: up to 5% of people in the U.S. and over 20% of people worldwide have a furrowed tongue. Despite the name, it's only slightly more common in men than in women. Scrotal tongue tends to increase in frequency and severity with age and is usually inherited.

As nasty as it sounds, scrotal tongue is usually a benign sign—unless bacteria fill in the grooves and cause *halitosis.* It can also be a sign of the rare condition *Miescher-Melkersson-Rosenthal syndrome,* which causes swelling of the lips. (See **Puffy Lips,** above.)

A SMOOTH TONGUE

Having a smooth tongue doesn't necessarily mean you're a smooth talker. Rather, if it's smooth and pale, it can be a sign of any one of several nutritional deficiencies, such as a lack of folic acid, vitamin B_{12}, or iron. As a result, the tongue loses its rough covering and may become tender and even shrink.

A smooth red tongue, however, can be a red flag for *pernicious anemia,* a fairly common and easily treatable vitamin B_{12} deficiency, or *malabsorption syndrome,* an intestinal disorder in which the body cannot adequately absorb nutrients.

If only a patch of your tongue is red or white and smooth, it may be a sign of *median rhomboid glossitis (MRG).* This bare spot looks much like a diamond or rhomboid, hence its name. It can be flat or raised and is devoid of both tongue hairs and taste buds. Usually found in the middle of the tongue toward the back, it can be quite small or can grow so large that it covers almost half of the tongue. An uncommon condition, MRG, also medically known as *central papillary atrophy,* is seen more frequently in men than in women.

People with MRG will sometimes get a *kissing lesion*—a red, irritated spot caused when the bare spot of the tongue rubs up against the soft palate. These spots may be mistaken for cancer, but they're not. They are, however, susceptible to thrush. (See **Burning, Tingling Lips or Mouth,** above.)

SIGNIFICANT FACT

Believe it or not, the longest tongue on record is a mere 3.74 inches (9.5 cm). This dubious distinction belongs to a British subject, according to the *Guinness Book of World Records.*

SPEAKING OF SIGNS

A sharp tongue is the only edged tool that grows keener with constant use.
—Washington Irving,
Rip Van Winkle, 1907

TRAVELING TONGUE PATCHES

Now you see it, now you don't. That's a pretty accurate description of a pretty weird condition called *geographic tongue* (aka *benign migratory glossitis*). The tip-off for geographic tongue is irregular patches of missing papillae that make the tongue look like a map, hence its name. The

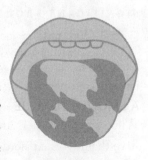

GEOGRAPHIC TONGUE

patches pop up in one place and then disappear, only to reappear on another part of the tongue. The spots may be white and rough or red and smooth.

Geographic tongue is a benign condition. Although its cause is unknown, it tends to run in families. It's usually painless, but some people have discomfort when eating spicy food.

TWITCHY TONGUE

Try keeping your tongue still while looking in a mirror at your open mouth. It's virtually impossible because a normal tongue will jerk and twitch. But a constantly quivering tongue may be a clue that you have *essential tremor (ET)*, a fairly common, slowly progressing, but usually not debilitating movement disorder that affects about 10 million people in the U.S. (See Chapter 7.)

A tongue tremor can also signal other movement disorders, such as Parkinson's disease or multiple sclerosis. In addition, twitchy tongue may be a reaction to medications used to treat anxiety and other psychological problems, or a telltale sign that you have a seriously overactive thyroid. (See Appendix I.)

TASTE DISORDERS

Our ability to taste depends not only on our taste buds, but also on the movement of our tongues. By pushing food around our mouths, our tongues spread food over our taste buds.

Our sense of taste is strongly wedded to our sense of smell. (See Chapter 4.) Indeed, these senses are so co-dependent that the loss of one often results in the loss of the other.

> **SIGNIFICANT FACT**
>
> ⚠ The taste of food is determined not only by its flavor but also by its texture, temperature, and smell.

While smell disorders are more common—more than 3 million Americans have them—taste disorders affect almost 2 million.

DIMINISHED OR DISTORTED SENSE OF TASTE

Has the salsa at your favorite Mexican restaurant lost its bite? It may merely mean that there's a new cook in the kitchen. On the other hand, it could well be a sign that you're losing your sense of taste, or more specifically the ability to detect and differentiate flavors—a condition medically known as *hypogeusia.* But if the spicy salsa begins to taste more like smoked salmon, it could signal *dysgeusia,* a distorted sense of taste.

> **SIGNIFICANT FACT**
>
> ⚠ Taste buds on the tip of the tongue detect sweetness. Those on the sides of the tip detect saltiness, while the ones on the sides of the tongue detect sourness. And the taste buds at the back of the tongue detect bitterness.

As with losing our other senses, a diminished sense of taste can be a natural sign of aging. Fortunately, a total loss of taste (*ageusia*) is rare.

Both the loss of taste and taste distortions may be signs of an oral infection or irritation from braces or dentures. People who have facial nerve damage (as in Bell's palsy) or who have had a head trauma or radiation to the head or neck may also sense that their taste is lessened or altered.

> **SIGNIFICANT FACT**
>
> ⚠ Taste buds are not just on our tongues. They're also in our throats, pharynx, larynx, epiglottis, uvula, and part of the esophagus as well.

Taste disorders can be a reaction to many of the same drugs that distort the sense of smell (see Chapter 4) or dry out the mouth, and they can signal the same conditions that cause dry mouth—such as Sjögren's syndrome. (See **A Dry Mouth or Excessive Thirst,** above, and Appendix I.) Because food must be mixed and moistened with saliva to be tasted, the sense of taste can be diminished, distorted, or even lost completely when the mouth is too dry.

Taste disorders can be important clues to a vitamin A or B_3 (niacin) deficiency as well. Less commonly, they may signal diabetes, multiple sclerosis, liver disease, AIDS, or cancer.

Any loss of taste, even a partial one, can have serious repercussions.

People with diminished taste often oversalt and oversweeten their food, which can be dangerous if they suffer from hypertension or diabetes. For those of us who have a taste for the good life, life without the richness and variety of food may seem hardly worth living. Unfortunately, people who lose their sense of taste can become depressed.

WARNING SIGN

Loss of taste can be downright dangerous. Without the ability to taste, you can't tell if food's spoiled. This raises your risk of food poisoning.

A METALLIC OR TERRIBLE TASTE

Occasionally we all awaken with a horrible taste in our mouths. But if your toothbrush and mouthwash fail to slay that "dragon mouth" and it sometimes gets worse during the day, it may be a sign of *phantom tastes* or *phantogeusia,* the most common taste complaint. People with this condition taste things that aren't there.

SIGNIFICANT FACT

There are four basic tastes: sweet, salty, sour, and bitter. However, some scientists claim there's a fifth, which they call *umami.* Recently discovered, umami is the distinctive taste of meat, certain cheeses, and mushrooms.

Phantom tastes can be a sign of Bell's palsy and of **burning mouth syndrome** (aka **burning tongue syndrome**), a rare condition that tends to affect menopausal women (see **Supersensitive Taste,** below) and is thought to be caused by nerve damage. It can signal a viral infection and Sjögren's syndrome as well. (See **A Dry Mouth or Excessive Thirst,** above, and Appendix I.)

Most people with phantogeusia complain of having a metallic taste in their mouths, aptly known as *metallic phantogeusia.* This can be a reaction to certain medications, including antibiotics, antidepressants, antihypertensives, drugs used to treat kidney stones and rheumatoid arthritis, and some vitamins. It's also a common result of chemotherapy and radiation treatment. A metallic taste signals to some epileptics that a seizure may be coming on.

If your taste in music leans more toward heavy metal than light rock, the metallic taste may be an unexpected result of another one of the latest trends—tongue piercing with a small metal barbell. It can also be a tip-off that your tongue—or even your gums or nose—is bleeding. The iron in your blood gives off a metallic taste.

A metallic taste can be a warning sign that old metal dental fillings may be leaching into your mouth and it's time to get new ones. If your cavities are filled with several different metals (as many of

> **SIGNIFICANT FACT**
>
> The older you are, the more insensitive you are to taste: foods need to be 3 times sweeter, 4 times more sour, 7 times more bitter, and 11 times more salty for you to taste than when you were younger.

them are a combination of mercury, silver, and others), it's like having a mini battery in your mouth. The mixed metals create a chemical or electrical reaction that produces a metallic taste, or even a shock. The tinny taste can also signal dry mouth or that you're on an excessively high-protein, low-fat diet. (See **Bad Breath,** below.)

SUPERSENSITIVE TASTE

Do you tend to find coffee too bitter, desserts too sweet, Mexican food too hot, and broccoli just too nasty to eat? If so, you may be what doctors call a *supertaster.* While you might think it makes you special, scientists believe that as many 25% of people are supersensitive to taste— a condition medically known as *hypergeusia.* This is an inherited trait that endows you with more taste buds than other people have. Women are more likely to be supertasters than men, and more South Americans, Africans, and Asians are supertasters than people of other regions.

> **SIGNIFICANT FACT**
>
> You can actually count your own taste buds. Dip a cotton swab into blue food coloring and coat the front of your tongue with the dye. Move your tongue around to spread the dye. Using a magnifying glass, count the blue-dyed taste buds in an area the size of a paper punch hole. If there are more than 20, you're a supertaster. If there are 4 to 6, you're a nontaster. Anything in between means you're just plain normal.

Because supertasters tend to shun strong-tasting foods, such as Brussels sprouts and cauliflower, they may lack adequate amounts of antioxidants and other important nutrients found in these vegetables.

Interestingly, people who are hypersensitive to taste are often hypersensitive to pain as well. Supersensitive taste may be a sign of *burning mouth syndrome* (see **A Metallic or Terrible Taste,** above), which is caused by nerve damage from a viral infection, hormonal changes, or both.

SIGNIFICANT FACT

Taste and smell cells are the only sensory cells that are replaced throughout a person's lifetime. Taste cells last about 10 days and are then replaced.

But there is an upside. Supertasters are less likely to smoke or abuse alcohol than others. And while your picky tastes may make dinner parties a nightmare for both you and your host, there's a good chance that you'll be a lot thinner than your fellow guests.

BAD BREATH

While our mouths have the power to please, they're also rife with ways to embarrass. And it's not just the ridiculous things we might say. Take bad breath, for example. It can take your—or someone else's—breath away! Unfortunately, we may not even realize we have bad breath until the humiliating moment when a friend or lover points it out to us.

SIGNIFICANT FACT

While foul breath can be a dead giveaway that someone's a smoker, it may someday save that smoker's life. Breath contains DNA, and researchers have found that smokers' breath can reveal DNA changes linked to lung cancer. The hope is that breath analysis will help detect lung cancer early in smokers and predict which of them are at high risk for this killer disease.

Bad breath can merely be a lingering sign of a garlic- or onion-rich diet. But chronic bad breath—medically known as *halitosis* or *fetororis*—is more often a sign of smoking or chewing tobacco and having poor dental hygiene. It can also signal that something is going terribly awry in your mouth, such as an abscessed or impacted tooth or a

gum, mouth, or tongue disease. About 85% of cases of bad breath originate in the mouth itself. The gastrointestinal or respiratory tracts are responsible for the rest.

If you suffer from noxious morning breath, it may be a sign of dry
mouth, which can result from
breathing through your mouth at
night from any of a number of medications and from certain disorders.
(See **A Dry Mouth or Excessive
Thirst,** above.)

SIGNIFICANT FACT

The body often shields itself
from its own foul odors. While
others may notice, there's a
good chance we won't smell our own
stinky breath.

Halitosis can signal postnasal
drip, strep throat, tonsillitis, sinus infection, or other respiratory tract conditions. It's also a major sign of *tonsilloliths* (aka *tonsil stones*)—small,
whitish, foul-smelling globules of food particles, dried mucus, and bacteria that lodge in the folds of the tonsils. Having enlarged, deep-creviced
tonsils or recurrent bouts of tonsillitis encourages the nasty buildup of
such debris. People who have these unsavory stones sometimes poke
them out with cotton swabs or sharp objects, but they usually come back.

Foul breath can also signal serious lung, kidney, and liver diseases.
Occasionally, it's a sign of certain
intestinal and digestive disorders,
including constipation, indigestion,
and gastric ulcers. Any condition
that causes frequent vomiting, including bulimia (see **Fecal Breath,**
below), can lead to bad breath.

SIGNIFICANT FACT

Your dog may be your best
friend in more ways than one.
A recent study found that
dogs can be trained to sniff out cancer by
smelling a person's breath. In fact, some
clever canines are such good diagnosti-
cians that they can learn to distinguish
between lung and breast cancer.

Stomach-related bad breath is actually fairly uncommon, but halitosis is reaching epidemic proportions among some dieters. It can, in fact,
be a telltale sign that someone is on the Atkins diet or another low-
carbohydrate, high-fat, high-protein diet. In fact, as many as two-thirds of
people on these diets suffer from bad breath, so they may lose friends as
well as weight. Their stinky breath is actually a sign that their body is
breaking down fat into *ketones* and going into a condition called *ketosis*
(elevated levels of ketones). Ketosis is considered a good sign for losing

weight, but it can lead to *acidosis,* an imbalance between the acids and alkalis in the blood, which is a serious condition that increases the risk of osteoporosis and kidney stones or worse. (See **Sweet, Fruity Breath,** below.)

WARNING SIGN

Bad breath—particularly in people who are very thin and/or obsessed with dieting—may be a tip-off that they're bulimic.

SWEET, FRUITY BREATH

When someone tells you your breath smells sweet, they may not just be sweet-talking you—they may, in fact, be saving your life. Sweet or fruity breath, or breath that has a sweet chemical or acetone (like nail polish remover) smell, can be a serious warning sign that you have diabetes and that your blood sugar is dangerously out of control. Medically known as *diabetic acidosis* or *diabetic ketoacidosis,* this is a medical emergency. If your blood sugar isn't promptly regulated, coma and death may follow.

SIGN OF THE TIMES

Bad breath was considered a serious disorder in the Talmud, the ancient Jewish scripture. Holy men with halitosis were forbidden to carry out holy rites. Bad breath was even considered grounds for divorce, a law that still exists in Israel today.

WARNING SIGN

When their blood sugar is out of control, diabetics may have a distinctive breath odor that smells like alcohol. Because low blood sugar can cause diabetics to stagger, they may be mistaken for being drunk and not receive the immediate medical help they need.

GARLIC BREATH

Does your mouth smell like garlic even when you haven't eaten any? If so, it may be a sign of *selenium toxicity* (aka *selenosis*). While an important antioxidant, selenium should not be taken in very large doses. In addition to supplements, it's found in nuts (especially Brazil nuts), meat, seafood, and—not surprisingly—garlic. But you'd be hard pressed to eat so much garlic—or any other selenium-containing food—to cause this problem.

Tooth discoloration and decay, skin discoloration, hair loss, nail problems, listlessness, and irritability are other signs of excess selenium. Selenosis can lead to neurological damage and in extreme cases result in lung disease, cirrhosis of the liver, and even death.

SIGNIFICANT FACT

Approximately 40 million Americans suffer from bad breath.

DANGER SIGN

Although very rare, garlic breath can be a dead giveaway of arsenic poisoning, especially if the person also complains of a metallic taste. This is a medical emergency.

URINE- OR AMMONIA-SMELLING BREATH

Breath that smells like pee or window cleaner is hard to ignore, at least by others. And that's a good thing. Urine- or ammonia-smelling breath can be a warning sign of kidney disease or even life-threatening chronic kidney failure. Because people with diabetes or hypertension are at increased risk for kidney disease, they should be on the lookout for this unpleasant warning sign.

SIGN OF THE TIMES

Hippocrates, the ancient Greek physician, had a distaste for women with bad breath. He recommended that all young women do the following to keep their breaths fresh: separately burn the head of a hare and three mice, mix the results with pulverized marble and apply to teeth and gums, and then rinse the mouth with dill seed, anise, and myrtle soaked in white wine.

FISHY BREATH

Did your last conversation with a co-worker smell fishy? Not what was said, but literally? A breath that smells distinctly like fish may be an all-too-obvious sign that your colleague is taking a lot of fish oil supplements for the omega-3 fatty acids. But it may also be a serious danger sign of kidney failure.

FECAL BREATH

If people say you have shitty breath, don't be too quick to punch them in the mouth. Fecal breath can signal conditions that, not surprisingly, are related to the stomach and digestion. For example, it can signal *gastroesophageal reflux disease* (aka *GERD* or *acid reflux*), a condition in which stomach acid backs up into the esophagus (see Chapters 6 and 8). Fecal breath can also be a sign of a scary-sounding and controversial condition called *intestinal permeability* (aka *leaky gut syndrome*), which is thought to be a quite common disorder in which the intestinal lining becomes overly porous. As the theory goes, toxins and undigested food leak into the bloodstream, which can trigger food allergies and autoimmune diseases.

> ### SIGN OF THE TIMES
>
> In 1921, the Listerine Company launched an advertising campaign to help boost the sale of their liquid antiseptic. They coined the term *halitosis* and sold their product as a mouthwash. It worked—both the new term and the product caught on. Annual sales jumped from $100,000 to over $4 million in just 6 years!

In addition, fecal breath can be a telltale sign of a bowel obstruction, which can be a medical emergency, or of repeated bouts of vomiting from bulimia. And like other forms of halitosis, fecal breath can signal serious respiratory and lung problems.

TEETH

You may think that your teeth are supposed to be pearly white, but actually they come in an assortment of colors, and not just because you don't brush them. Tooth enamel is translucent, so our teeth take on the color of the *dentin*, a hard yel-

> ### SPEAKING OF SIGNS
>
> *Teeth placed before the tongue give good advice.*
>
> —Italian proverb

low substance, inside them. The color of our teeth can tell us a lot about what goes on inside our bodies. In addition, tooth enamel can become stained from whatever we put in our mouths.

YELLOW-BROWN TEETH

If you're older and notice that your teeth are yellowing or becoming darker, it may be an unpleasant sign of aging. At any age it may be a tell-tale sign that you're a smoker or a heavy coffee, tea, or cola drinker.

GREENISH OR METALLIC-COLORED TEETH

Teeth stained green, bluish green, or brown can be a sign that you've been overexposed to some metals. This may have happened at work or during a dental procedure. The hue depends on the metal or the chemical reaction it has with the germs in your mouth. Exposure to iron, manganese, and silver may stain the teeth black, for example. Mercury and lead dust can leave a blue-green stain, while copper and nickel can turn teeth green to blue-green. Inhaling certain fumes, such as chromic acid, will stain teeth a deep orange. And overexposure to iodine solution and spending a lot of time in chlorinated pools can stain teeth brown.

SIGN OF THE TIMES

Although a New Orleans dentist is credited with inventing dental floss in the 19th century, dental floss and toothpicks have been found in the teeth of prehistoric humans. More recently, two creative uses for dental floss have surfaced: cutting cheesecake and making a makeshift rope. In 1994 a prisoner fashioned rope out of floss he saved up, thus escaping from a West Virginia penitentiary.

BLUISH GRAY TEETH

Many people are aware that taking the antibiotic tetracycline during pregnancy can cause a baby's teeth to come in discolored. The discoloration can also happen to children who take tetracycline when their permanent teeth are forming. Bluish gray stains in an adult may, however, be a sign of long-term use of minocycline, a type of tetracycline often prescribed to treat acne and rheumatoid arthritis. Gray teeth can also be a telltale sign of damaged dentin from a previous infection.

WARNING SIGN

While an aspirin a day may protect your heart, it may be bad for your teeth. Indeed, tooth erosion can be a sign that you've been sucking or chewing, rather than swallowing, the aspirin. When dissolved in the mouth, aspirin can, over time, wear away the teeth's protective enamel.

SPOTTED TEETH

Are your teeth more speckled than evenly colored? If so, it may be a sign of *enamel fluorosis,* an overexposure to fluoride from fluorinated drinking water, toothpaste, and oral rinses. In mild cases, the spots are small, whitish, and opaque. As the problem gets worse, the spots become brown and the teeth look mottled. While this condition often starts during childhood when developing teeth are exposed to too much fluoride, the brown stains and pitting are not usually spotted until much later. Although spotted teeth are cosmetically unappealing, they usually are a benign sign. However, these spots can be the earliest warning sign of fluoride poisoning, which can be life-threatening.

SIGN OF THE TIMES

In the first century B.C., the Roman author and philosopher Pliny the Elder recommended goat feet ashes to clean teeth. If you think that was gross, here's another popular teeth-cleaning solution of the time: take feces from a sheep's tail, roll it up into a small ball, dry it, then pulverize it into a powder and rub on the teeth!

WARNING SIGN

Overindulging is not the only thing wine tasters have to worry about. Another common occupational hazard is the loss of the surface of their teeth. Over time, bathing the teeth in the acid-containing wine erodes tooth enamel.

BLACKISH TEETH

If you see someone with black, stained, and crumbling teeth and you're not watching *Pirates of the Caribbean,* it can be quite a chilling sight. And you should be alarmed. These are the hallmarks of *meth mouth,* a newly described condition. Within a year of methamphetamine abuse, a person can often be left with root stumps and mushy mounds of decay. The sugary drinks meth users down to relieve the dry mouth that the drug causes can worsen the tooth decay. Unfortunately, most people with meth mouth often lose their teeth—and sometimes even their lives.

SPEAKING OF SIGNS

White sugar, black teeth.
—Croatian proverb

INDENTED OR NOTCHED TEETH

If you have smooth indentations on your teeth, it may be a sign that you're eating too many oranges and lemons. Acid in these and other foods can wear down tooth enamel, causing *tooth erosion.*

A V-shaped notch at the bottom of your teeth near your gum line can be a sign of over-zealous brushing. Sometimes overuse of toothpicks can also cause these grooves, because you're actually digging through your teeth's protective enamel coating. But more likely these notches are a sign of teeth grinding—medically called **bruxism** (see **Cracked Teeth,** below).

SIGN OF THE TIMES

The Mayans believed that if a pregnant woman pocketed a comb in the folds of her skirt, her child would have crooked teeth.

SMOOTH, GLASSY-LOOKING TEETH

If your teeth—especially your back teeth—feel as smooth as glass, it may sound appealing, but, sorry to say, it's not a good sign. It may, indeed, be a warning sign of bone loss (*osteoporosis*). It can also be a telltale sign of the eating disorder bulimia. Repeated vomiting bathes teeth in stomach acid, eroding their protective enamel. In fact, nearly 90% of bulimics have signs of tooth erosion.

WARNING SIGNS

Mouth-related signs of eating disorders include:
- Swollen salivary glands
- Changes in tooth color, shape, and length
- Brittle teeth
- Translucent teeth
- Red, dry, cracked lips
- Bad breath

CRACKED TEETH

If you're among the 20% of adults who grind or clench their teeth during the day and the 8% of those who do it in their sleep, you may see or feel a fracture on your teeth. A fractured back tooth, which is especially common in people with silver fillings, is often a sign of *bruxism,* which affects men and women equally. (See Chapter 6.) Bruxism is actually more destructive to teeth than cavities. Because protective tooth enamel can be worn down during teeth grinding and clenching, teeth can become very sensitive as well. Even false teeth can bear the signs of teeth grinding and clenching. And grinding or clenching teeth, whether awake or asleep, can often lead to jaw problems, such as *temporomandibular joint disorder (TMJ).* (See Chapter 6.)

SPEAKING OF SIGNS

A knife is the tooth of the old; the tooth is the oldest knife.

—Finnish proverb

SPEAKING OF SIGNS

Hot things, sharp things, sweet things, cold things—all rot the teeth, and make them look like old things.

—Benjamin Franklin,
Poor Richard's Almanac

SIGNING OFF

Many different specialists can evaluate and treat disorders and diseases of the lips and mouth. Which one you discuss your problem with depends on the location and type of sign you have. Remember, if you have bleeding or pain, these are sure signs that need to be checked out quickly. Here are just a few of the health care professionals you may be talking to when it comes to your lips, mouth, and teeth:

- *Dental hygienist:* A health care professional licensed in dental hygiene who specializes in preventing tooth and gum disease. In addition to cleaning teeth, dental hygienists are trained to evaluate the teeth, gums, and mouth for abnormalities.
- *Dentist:* A specialist with a Doctor of Dental Surgery (DDS) or Doctor of Medical Dentistry (DMD) degree. (These degrees and training are the same.) Dentists can treat periodontal disease as part of overall dental care.
- *Dermatologist:* A medical doctor who has been trained in diagnosing and treating skin diseases.
- *Endodontist (endodontologist):* A dentist who specializes in root canal procedures, diagnosing and managing oral/facial pain, and other clinical procedures related to the dental pulp (soft inner tissues of the teeth).
- *Oral surgeon:* A dentist with special training in surgery of the mouth and jaw.
- *Otolaryngologist* (also known as *otorhinolaryngologist*): A medical doctor who specializes in diagnosing and treating ear, nose, and throat diseases and disorders.
- *Periodontist:* A DDS or DMD specializing in diagnosing, treating, and preventing gum disease.

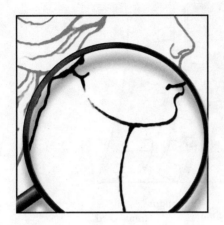

CHAPTER 6

TELLING THE TRUTH

Your Throat, Voice, Neck, and Jaw

I've tried several varieties of sex. The conventional position makes me claustrophobic and the others give me a stiff neck or lockjaw.

—ACTRESS TALLULAH BANKHEAD

Our head houses not only our senses but also some of the most sensual and beautiful parts of our bodies. However, with the exception of such long-necked beauties as Queen Nefertiti and Audrey Hepburn, the throat, jaw, and neck don't usually merit much aesthetic attention. Indeed, collars, scarves, and necklaces were designed to cover up or enhance these often unremarkable and sometimes unattractive body parts. Nonetheless, they do play important roles: they are our personal food processors, they help us speak the words and sing the songs we and others love to hear, and last but not least, our throat, jaw, and neck can speak volumes about our state of health and illness.

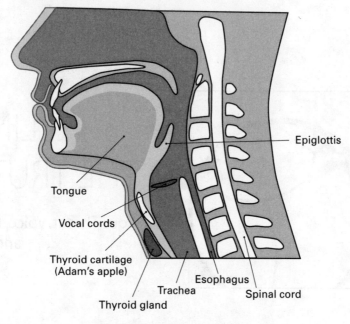

Epiglottis

Tongue

Vocal cords

Thyroid cartilage
(Adam's apple)

Esophagus

Trachea

Spinal cord

Thyroid gland

THROAT AND NECK ANATOMY

NECK, THROAT, AND JAW

LUMPS ON THE FRONT OF THE NECK

If you have a lump on your throat that's always been there, it's most likely your Adam's apple. The Adam's apple is actually thyroid cartilage, which is the largest of the five cartilages that make up the voice box (larynx). The thyroid cartilage is not the same thing as the thyroid gland, although they're very near each other.

> **SIGN OF THE TIMES**
>
> The Adam's apple is so called because it was believed that a piece of the forbidden fruit got caught in Adam's throat.

Even Eves have Adam's apples, but they're usually smaller than those in men. The Adam's apple is found on the front of the neck and is perfectly normal. It's the lumps farther down your neck or those on the side of your neck that you need to heed. Any lump or nodule on the neck can signal a tumor, which may or may not be cancerous.

A lump below your Adam's apple may be a *goiter,* an enlarged thyroid gland, which is a sign of thyroid disease.

The American Association of Clinical Endocrinologists has devised The Thyroid Neck Check for detecting a goiter.

- Stand in front of a mirror.
- Stretch the neck back.
- Swallow some water.
- Look for enlargement in the neck (below the Adam's apple, above the collarbone).
- If you see one, feel the area to confirm enlargement or bump.
- If you feel one, consult a doctor.

The thyroid is a small, butterfly-shaped gland in your neck that produces *thyroxin* (also spelled *thyroxine),* the hormone that controls metabolism. (Although only about 2 inches across, the thyroid is the largest gland in our body.) Our bodies need iodine to manufacture this vital hormone, and in the past, most goiters were signs of iodine deficiency. With the introduction of iodized salt in the 1920s, iodine-deficiency goiters became extremely rare in the United States and many other countries.

Today, most goiters in the United States are telltale signs of thyroid disease. Paradoxically, a goiter may signal either too much thyroid hormone (*hyperthyroidism*) or too little (*hypothyroidism*). (See Appendix I.) Because goiters can grow slowly and are usually painless, they sometimes go unnoticed until they become so large that your shirt collar feels tight.

Goiters can sometimes signal a pregnancy. During pregnancy, the thyroid gland often becomes enlarged, resulting in a goiter and sometimes thyroid disease. Indeed, a goiter in some new mothers may signal a form of autoimmune hypothyroidism called *Hashimoto's disease.* This is the most common type of hypothyroidism, and women—pregnant

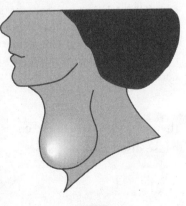

GOITER

or otherwise—are three times more likely than men to develop it. Like other forms of hypothyroidism, it can cause weight gain, cold intolerance, dry skin and hair, and constipation. Hypothyroidism is easily treated, and sometimes, along with the goiter, it can even disappear on its own.

SIGNIFICANT FACT

One-third of women and children in the world suffer from iodine deficiency, the most common cause of goiter. Iodine deficiency is also the leading cause of preventable mental retardation in children.

More commonly, however, a goiter is a sign of Graves' disease (see Chapter 2), an autoimmune hyperthyroid disorder. In spite of its name, Graves' disease is not normally a grave condition if treated. However, a person with Graves' disease (or any other type of hyperthyroidism) can develop *thyrotoxicosis*, very high levels of thyroid hormones. If left untreated, it can progress to a *thyroid storm* (aka *thyrotoxic crisis*), which can cause congestive heart failure and death.

A goiter can also be your body's way of saying that you're eating too many foods known as *goitrogens*. Excess consumption of goitrogens can promote goiters—medically referred to as *sporadic goiters*—by interfering with your body's ability to absorb iodine. The most common goitrogenic culprits are soybeans, soy products, and cruciferous vegetables such as cabbage, Brussels sprouts, and broccoli. Interestingly, a goiter can be a sign that you're consuming too much iodine itself, from either food or supplements.

SIGN OF THE TIMES

In the early 20th century, goiters were very common in a section of the United States referred to as the "goiter belt." These areas, which were remote from the sea, included the Midwest, Great Lakes region, Appalachia, and other mountainous areas. Without iodine-rich soil, sea salt, seafood, or seaweed, most people in these regions couldn't get the iodine they needed for their thyroid glands to function properly.

Goiters can occasionally signal thyroid cancer. In those cases the goiter is often large, hard, and may cause discomfort or pain.

LUMPS ELSEWHERE ON THE NECK

If a lump appears on the back of your neck, you may not be aware of it until someone points it out to you. A round or oval painless lump on the back of the neck may be a sign of a *lipoma*, a soft, rubbery, movable fatty tumor under the skin. (See Chapter 9.) They're the most common noncancerous soft-tissue tumor in adults and are most prevalent among women and overweight people. If they change size or appearance, however, they may be cancerous.

A lump on the nape of your neck can be also be a sign of a *sebaceous cyst* (aka *epidermal*, *epidermoid*, or *keratin* cyst). Sebaceous cysts are also soft, movable, and painless. (See Chapter 9.) But unlike lipomas, they usually have an indentation or dark spot in the middle. These cysts are actually swollen hair follicles that become filled with gross-smelling, cheesy, pasty substances including the protein *keratin*, which sometimes leaks out. Sebaceous cysts may sometimes show up on the face and trunk and are benign. Ranging in size from about ¼ inch to over 2 inches, they can grow even larger or disappear on their own. And they may become infected and/or grow so big, tender, and inflamed that they need to be drained or removed.

SIGNIFICANT FACT

More than 40,000 cases of cancers of the head and neck are diagnosed each year in the United States. Heavy drinkers and smokers are at highest risk. And the combination of both these unhealthy habits is synergistic, dramatically increasing the cancer risk.

SIGN OF THE TIMES

A popular old Nebraskan folk cure for goiters involved wrapping a snake around the neck. It was believed that as the snake slithered away, so would the goiter.

DANGER SIGN

While sebaceous cysts, lipomas, and other skin growths are most often benign, it's important to have any new or changing skin growth on your body checked out by a dermatologist to rule out cancer.

A painless, slow-growing, but movable lump on the side of your neck or under the chin may signal a salivary gland tumor—medically known as *submandibular tumor*. These tumors are actually blocked salivary glands and can pop up almost anywhere on the face and neck and in the mouth. The good news is that these growths, like lipomas, are usually not cancerous. If, however, you have a nonmovable lump along with such signs as nerve weakness, numbness, or hoarseness, it may signal cancer.

WARNING SIGN

A swollen salivary gland that becomes painful, grows rapidly, can't be moved around under the skin, or is accompanied by hoarseness may be a malignant tumor.

A painless, hard lymph node on the side of your neck behind your jawbone can be an early warning sign of *lymphoma*, including *Hodgkin's disease* and *non-Hodgkin's lymphoma*. Both are rare forms of cancer of the lymph nodes. Non-Hodgkin's lymphoma accounts for about 5% of cancers in the United States and is mostly found in adults around age 60. Hodgkin's is much rarer and primarily affects younger people between the ages of 15 and 35. Although both conditions can be fatal, they can be treated successfully if caught early.

SIGNIFICANT FACT

Lymph nodes (aka lymph glands) are small, bean-shaped infection fighters that keep the body healthy by filtering out or trapping bacteria, viruses, cancer cells, and other toxic substances. About one-third of the 500 to 600 lymph nodes in the body are on the sides of the neck and on the throat. Others are found in the groin, chest, abdomen, and armpits.

Enlarged lymph nodes in the neck can also signal cancer of the thyroid, throat, or even gastrointestinal tract.

A LUMP IN THE THROAT

Most of us have had the uncomfortable feeling of a lump in our throat—that choked-up sensation when we're trying to hold back tears. But constantly feeling like you have a lump in your throat that swallowing doesn't relieve may be what's medically known as the *globus sensation*. This condition used to be called *globus hystericus* because it was thought to be a sign of a psychological rather than a physical problem. It mainly affects women, hence the medical term *hystericus,* which is Latin for "of the womb."

Globus may in fact be a sign of anxiety. However, it can also signal one of the most common types of reflux, *gastrointestinal reflux disease (GERD)*. (See **A Hoarse, Raspy Voice,** below.) It could also be due to hypothyroidism or to esophageal or throat problems. In rare cases, the feeling of a lump in the throat may be a warning sign of a tumor in the esophagus or larynx.

SPEAKING OF SIGNS

A poem begins with a lump in the throat.

—Robert Frost

SIGN OF THE TIMES

In the past, the term *hystericus* was used to describe disorders that primarily affected women and were thought to be of psychological origin. Indeed, Freud and some of his followers believed that *globus hystericus,* which is rarely seen in men, signified fear of or guilt about sex, especially oral sex.

A LUMP ON THE JAW

You look in the mirror one morning and staring you back is the mother of all pimples. While you may think this is a sign of regression to your acne-filled days of puberty, what it may actually signal is *lumpy jaw* or *actinomycosis*—a chronic infection that causes an abscess. Sometimes people with these infections have other neck and throat signs, including hoarseness. Lumpy jaw can be more than a blight on your social life. If untreated, the infection can go to your brain.

CLICKING JAW

Your breakfast cereal may snap, crackle, or pop, but if your jaw does the same whenever you bite into your food or yawn, you might have one of the most common signs of the very common condition *temporomandibular joint disorder (TMJ)*. (See Chapter 5.) Other TMJ signs may include ringing or pain in the ears, sensitive teeth, jaw locking, and pain. Clicking can also signal that your teeth are misaligned (*malocclusion*). Not surprisingly, if you've been whacked in the face, you could wind up with a jaw that clicks.

STIFF JAW

If you have difficulty opening your mouth, your partner might consider it a blessing. But this may, in fact, be a condition known medically as *trismus*, which can be more than an inconvenience when trying to talk or eat. Trismus can start suddenly or develop slowly. It's another common sign of TMJ. (See **Clicking Jaw**, above.) It can also signal some more serious problems such as *tetanus* (aka *lockjaw*), a tumor, or several autoimmune disorders, including *lupus* (see Appendix I) or *scleroderma*. (See Chapter 9.) And people who've had a face or jaw injury or who've undergone head and neck radiation therapy sometimes have difficulty opening their mouths completely.

If your jaw feels stiff and you can't move it from side to side, it may be a serious sign of oral cancer. (See Chapter 5.) Swelling can be another jaw sign of cancer of the mouth or other parts of the head and neck. But the swelling can be so subtle that you may not recognize it until you have trouble chewing. People with false teeth may notice that their dentures don't fit as well as before.

WARNING SIGN

Recently, a rare but very serious condition, *osteonecrosis of the jaw* (literally, death of the jawbone), has been linked to the bone-building drugs bisphosphonates especially when used to treat some cancer-related bone complications. While these drugs are also commonly prescribed to prevent and treat *osteopenia* and *osteoporosis* (bone loss), osteonecrosis of the jaw has occurred only rarely with these uses.

RECEDING OR THRUSTING CHIN

A receding hairline can be covered with a hat, but a receding chin is harder to hide. Unfortunately, it can be more than a cosmetic concern; it can be a sign of chronic TMJ. (See **Stiff Jaw** and **Clicking Jaw,** above.) The inflamed, swollen jaw muscles can lose their grip; as a result, the jaw recedes.

If you've ever seen someone whose chin keeps thrusting out while they blink their eyes repeatedly, it's likely a sign of *Meige's syndrome,* a rare neurological movement disorder. (See Chapter 2.) Some people with Meige's also have *laryngeal dysphonia,* which causes their voice to sound strained and strangled, or like a staticky radio. (See **Voice Signs,** below.)

SIGN OF THE TIMES

The Habsburg family, which ruled much of Europe from the 10th century to the 20th, was famous for their protruding lips and prominent jaws (dubbed the "Habsburg jaw"). These unattractive family traits were signs of royal inbreeding. One family member—17th-century Holy Roman Emperor Leopold I—had such a prominent jaw that he was nicknamed "The Hogmouth."

FREQUENT YAWNING

If you're with someone who starts yawning, you may think it's a sign of boredom. You may be right and may even join in. Indeed, yawning has long been known to be contagious.

People yawn for a variety of other reasons, such as fatigue. While we might yawn when we're sleepy, we yawn just as much when we first awaken—even after a good night's sleep.

Theories concerning yawning abound. Some scientists believe that yawning helps us become more alert by taking in oxygen; others say it's due to changes in emotion-related brain chemicals; still others think it helps regulate body temperature. They all tend to agree, however, that yawning does boost blood pressure and heart rate. According to anecdotal evidence, some athletes have been known to habitually yawn before a competition and paratroopers to do so before a jump.

Most of the time, yawning is a benign, if rather boring, activity. Sometimes, however, yawning can forewarn of a type of fainting—medically known as *vasovagal syncope*—the kind we usually associate with fainting from fear.

And sometimes yawning can be a wake-up call that we may have a serious medical condition. Although the reasons are unknown, people with some neurological conditions—including *multiple sclerosis* and *amyotropic lateral sclerosis (ALS)*, commonly called *Lou Gehrig's disease*—often yawn excessively. Sometimes frequent yawning is a reaction to radiation therapy for cancer as well as drugs to treat *Parkinson's disease*. Some antidepressants, such as paroxetine (Paxil) and sertraline (Zoloft), can also cause excessive yawning. Interestingly, schizophrenics tend to yawn less frequently than others.

> ### SIGNIFICANT FACT
>
> Just about all vertebrates yawn. In fact, human fetuses start yawning at about 11 weeks. From start to finish a yawn takes about 6 seconds.

> ### SIGNIFICANT FACT
>
> A recent psychiatric journal reported that several patients had an unusual, albeit pleasurable, reaction to the antidepressant clomipramine. For them, yawning is anything but a snore—every time they yawn they have a spontaneous orgasm. One woman became extremely adept at having orgasms by yawning. On the other hand, one man found the experience a big inconvenience—he continuously had to wear a condom.

> ### SPEAKING OF SIGNS
>
> *Life is too short, and the time we waste in yawning never can be regained.*
>
> —Stendhal, 19th-century French writer

EXCESSIVE HICCUPPING

If you're with someone who starts hiccupping uncontrollably, you may find it funny at first, then annoying—especially if your companion has been drinking a lot. Hiccups are, in fact, a common, telltale sign of excessive drinking.

Hiccups (also spelled hiccoughs) are medically known as *singultus,* which comes from the Latin *singult,* meaning "the act of catching one's breath while sobbing." Hiccups are involuntary spasms of the diaphragm and they tend to occur when the level of carbon dioxide in the blood drops too low. Noxious fumes, smoking, and spicy foods or drinks can set off a

SIGN OF THE TIMES

 In 1988, Dr. Francis Fesmire hit upon an unusual cure for intractable hiccups. His patient had been hiccupping 30 times a minute for 72 hours. After trying every known remedy to no avail, the undaunted doctor decided to stimulate the vagus nerve by inserting his finger in the man's anus. This *digital rectal massage,* as it's medically known, worked. Fesmire is now promoting something more appealing—orgasms. They're tremendous stimulators of the vagus nerve, he explained.

bout. So can having a cold drink while eating a hot meal. In fact, hiccups may be your body's way of saying you're eating or drinking too much or too fast. One theory is that hiccups are reflexes that keep you from choking on food and beverages.

Most bouts of hiccupping are brief, lasting only a few minutes; but sometimes they can continue considerably longer. An attack that goes on for more than 2 or 3 hours is referred to as *persistent* or *protracted hiccups. Intractable hiccups* are usually defined as hiccups

SIGN OF THE TIMES

 The record for the longest lasting fit of hiccups goes to Charles Osborne of Iowa, who died in 1990 at the age of 96. His hiccups started after he slaughtered a hog, according to the *Guinness Book of World Records,* and they continued for 69 years.

lasting more than a month. Both types of hiccups are much more common in men than women. It's believed that persistent and intractable hiccups are caused by runaway electrical impulses in the *vagus nerve,* which runs from the brain stem to the abdomen and controls heart rate, stomach acid production, intestines, and throat muscles, among other key functions. They're also thought to be caused by irritation of the phrenic nerve, which is the motor nerve to the diaphragm that helps control breathing. In fact, the phrenic nerve used to be cut to stop uncontrolled hiccupping.

In general, if your partner has unrelenting hiccups that stop during sleep, it's apt to be a sign of stress or other intense emotions. But if your bedmate hiccups while sleeping, it's more likely to signal a physical problem.

Hiccupping can be a tip-off that you have a foreign body or growth in your ear, or suffer from GERD. (See **A Lump in the Throat,** above.) And long bouts of hiccups are known to both precede and follow fainting spells due to heart rhythm problems. In addition, more than one-third of patients who undergo chemotherapy complain of persistent hiccups.

SPEAKING OF SIGNS

Hold your breath, and if after you have done so for some time the hiccup is no better, then gargle with a little water, and if it still continues, tickle your nose with something and sneeze, and if you sneeze once or twice, even the most violent hiccup is sure to go.

—Eriximachus, physician to Aristophanes

STOP SIGNS

There are several home remedies for common hiccups. Many raise blood carbon dioxide levels or stimulate the vagus nerve to help it get back on track. The "cures" include:

- Holding your breath
- Breathing into a paper bag
- Pulling your tongue
- Rubbing your eyeballs
- Swallowing dry bread
- Eating crushed ice
- Eating a teaspoon of sugar
- Using smelling salts
- Drinking a glass of water quickly without breathing

Prolonged hiccups can also be a sign of *pneumonia, pleurisy* (an inflammation of the lungs), *peritonitis* (an infection of the abdominal cavity), *pericarditis* (an inflammation of the membrane surrounding the heart), and *pancreatitis* (an inflammation of the pancreas). They can also signal chronic kidney disease or failure, as well as an infection or tumor in the diaphragm, esophagus, or lungs. Rarely, persistent or intractable hiccups can be a danger sign of a stroke or brain tumor, either of which can disrupt the brain's breathing center.

CHRONIC COUGHING

If you seem to always be hacking away but feel fine and don't smoke, don't chalk it up to just an annoying habit. Persistent coughing is a common reaction to ACE (angiotensin-converting enzyme) inhibitors, a type of blood pressure medication. And it can be a sign of postnasal drip, allergies, asthma, or GERD. (See **A Hoarse, Raspy Voice,** below.) More important, it can signal *chronic obstructive pulmonary disease (COPD),* a debilitating and

> **SIGNIFICANT FACT**
>
> Lung cancer is the leading cause of cancer deaths in the United States among both men and women. Indeed, more women die each year from lung cancer than from breast, ovarian, and uterine cancer combined.

potentially deadly lung disorder in which airflow to and from the lungs is disrupted. There are two main types of COPD: *chronic bronchitis* and *emphysema.* COPD affects approximately 28 million people in the United States alone; half of them are undiagnosed. Although COPD is incurable, treatments may help relieve some of its symptoms, prevent complications, and prolong life.

Of course, if you are or were a smoker—or live with one—there's a chance that your coughing is a warning sign not only of COPD but of lung or throat cancer as well. Smoking is the primary cause of all these conditions. Unfortunately, frequent coughing can be a sign of both COPD and cancer even if you've never touched a cigarette in your life.

COLORED PHLEGM

Coughing up great globs of mucus—or *phlegm,* as it's medically known—can be quite gross. It can be revealing as well. (Phlegm is sometimes referred to as *sputum,* which is actually the mixture of phlegm with saliva.) Regardless of what it's called, in a healthy person it's usually clear or whitish. If, however, your phlegm is clear but very sticky, it may signal asthma. If you're bringing up a lot of clear phlegm, it's most likely from a viral infection. But yellow, green, or brown phlegm likely signals a bacterial infection. Brown phlegm can be a sign that you smoke too much and may have lung damage. But if you're a smoker and you have a morning cough that produces clear sputum, you're not off the hook. It may be a very early warning sign of COPD. (See **Chronic Coughing,** above.) If your morning cough produces yellow or green sputum and you're short of breath, you may have an advanced case of COPD. If your phlegm is rust-colored or looks like it's streaked with blood, it may be a sign of *hemoptysis*—blood from an infection or tumor in the respiratory tract, including the nose, mouth, throat, esophagus, or lungs. Bleeding from the lungs can signal pneumonia or even more serious lung disorders including cancer. The blood-tinged sputum can also signal gastrointestinal bleeding, medically known as *pseudohemoptysis.*

VOICE SIGNS

Our voices depend on a myriad of body parts to make even a simple sound—the vocal cords, lips, tongue, teeth, soft palate, throat, larynx, windpipe, lungs, diaphragm, and nose, to name a few. When something goes wrong with any one of these body parts, our voices can do more than complain. Their clarity, quality, and volume can often help pinpoint the problem.

SPEAKING OF SIGNS
The voice is nothing but beaten air.
—Seneca the Younger, ancient Greek philosopher and dramatist

About 7.5 million people in the United States have voice problems, medically known as *dysphonia*. Like many body signs, voice changes can be a common but benign sign of aging. As we age, our lung tissue loses elasticity, and our respiratory and other muscles weaken or stiffen, in part because of hormonal changes. Men often speak at a higher pitch as they age, perhaps because their estrogen levels tend to rise, and older women tend to notice that their voices deepen because their estrogen levels fall. But these and other vocal changes can be telling us that something else is going on in our bodies.

SPEAKING OF SIGNS

The human voice is the organ of the soul.

—Henry Wadsworth Longfellow

A HOARSE, RASPY VOICE

Does your voice often sound gravelly when you try to speak? A husky voice on a man—or even a woman—can sound sexy (think Marlene Dietrich). But most of us find a raspy or gravelly voice irritating to have...and to hear.

SIGN OF THE TIMES

Throughout his presidency, and still today, Bill Clinton has been plagued with a hoarse voice. It's been attributed to everything from allergies and asthma to voice overuse.

An occasional bout of hoarseness—medically known as *laryngitis*—is normally a sign of nothing more serious than a cold, allergy, or postnasal drip. But it may also signal a more serious respiratory tract infection. And hoarseness can be a wake-up call that you've been straining your voice—or, more accurately, your vocal cords (aka vocal folds). Although shouting and yelling are prime perpetrators of laryngitis, you don't necessarily have to be a screamer to become hoarse. Repeated whispering and throat clearing can be culprits. And if you're living with someone who's hard of hearing, your voice may become hoarse from speaking in a louder-than-normal tone. Or your husky voice may be a sign that you, too, are getting older.

If your raspy voice lingers longer than two weeks, it's definitely worth voicing your concern. It can be a sign of one of two kinds of reflux, either *gastroesophageal reflux disease* (*GERD*) or *reflux laryngitis,* aka *laryngopharyngeal reflux (LPR)*. In GERD, stomach acid backs up into the esophagus, while in LPR, the acid makes it all the way to the back of the throat. Morning hoarseness—especially along with heartburn and nausea—can be a sign of both types of reflux. Other signs include a bitter taste, a burning sensation, or the feeling of having something stuck in your throat. (See **A Lump in the Throat,** above.) Without treatment, reflux can result in sinus and ear infections, throat lesions, and *Barrett's esophagus,* a peptic ulcer in the lower esophagus, which can lead to esophageal cancer.

SPEAKING OF SIGNS

Screaming is bad for the voice, but good for the heart.

—Conor Oberst, American rock singer ("Bright Eyes") and composer

A deep, gravelly voice, especially in women, is often a dead giveaway of heavy smoking, now or in the past. Indeed, many women who smoke are mistaken for men over the phone. Whether you're a man or a woman, smoking can cause your vocal cords to thicken, giving you the characteristic "smoker's voice."

SIGNIFICANT FACT

GERD affects more than 60 million adult Americans. Men are about 2 times more likely than women to have it. The average age of people diagnosed with GERD is 60.

Smoker's voice is often a sign of *Reinke's edema,* a swelling of the vocal cords rarely seen in nonsmokers. Unfortunately, this sign is often overlooked in men because it's not unusual for them to have deep voices. It's a clear clue that smoking has already caused severe damage.

WARNING SIGN

Hoarseness is the hallmark of cancer of the vocal cords, and smoking is its main cause. If untreated, the cancer will grow and damage the larynx, causing speaking and breathing difficulties, and ultimately death. So not only should people with smoker's voice quit smoking, they should be examined periodically for precancerous and cancerous lesions.

Chronic hoarseness can also be a telltale sign of long-term heavy drinking. Excess alcohol, like smoke, can irritate the vocal cords as well as the mucous membranes in the mouth and throat.

A very husky voice can be evidence of a hormonal imbalance in either sex. In women, it can be a sign of a hormone disorder called *masculinization,* in which there are high levels of the male hormone androgen. (See Chapter 1.)

STOP SIGN

To protect your vocal cords and ward off hoarseness:
- Don't repeatedly clear your throat.
- Don't scream or whisper unless absolutely necessary.
- Avoid caffeinated drinks, alcohol, and dairy products.
- Drink lots of water.

If you live in an industrial town, your raspy voice may be telling you that environmental irritants and pollutants are lurking about. Huskiness can also be a reaction to radiation therapy as well as to certain medicines. The most common culprits are blood thinners, antihypertensives, antihistamines, steroids, asthma medicines, antidepressants, diuretics, and high doses of vitamin C.

A hoarse voice may also signal *iron deficiency anemia,* as well as a host of serious autoimmune conditions including *myasthenia gravis, rheumatoid arthritis, Sjögren's syndrome,* and *sarcoidosis.* (See Appendix I.) And a hoarse voice in the morning (aka morning voice) is a common sign of hypothyroidism. (See Appendix I.) Chronic hoarseness can also be a warning sign of benign or malignant growths on the vocal cords, throat, mouth, or neck. Although these growths are much more common in smokers, nonsmokers can get them as well.

SIGN OF THE TIMES

A popular myth in China is that if a pregnant woman eats chicken or rabbit, her baby will develop a hoarse voice.

A SPORADICALLY HOARSE VOICE

If you sometimes get hoarse, have trouble breathing—that "can't catch your breath" feeling—cough, and wheeze, you may worry that you have asthma. But these signs may be pointing to a little-known medical condition called *vocal cord dysfunction (VCD)*. Indeed, VCD is often misdiagnosed as asthma, especially when people turn up in the emergency room with other common asthma-like signs such as a tightening in the chest and turning blue. As its name implies, VCD results when a person's vocal cords don't open and close properly to let air in and out during speech. A VCD attack can be triggered by nasal problems or either GERD or LPR. (See **A Hoarse, Raspy Voice,** above.) VCD can also signal that you're being exposed to environmental or occupational pollutants.

SIGNIFICANT FACT

The vocal cords vibrate 80 to 400 times per second.

FREQUENT THROAT CLEARING

Do you constantly clear your throat? This may be a bad habit you acquired after a persistent cough or a long bout of laryngitis. Frequent throat clearing may also be the sign of anxiety and nervousness or of a tic or other movement disorder. As with hoarseness, it can also be an important clue that you have chronic postnasal drip or GERD. (See **A Hoarse, Raspy Voice,** above.)

STOP SIGN

When you feel the urge to clear your throat, sip water or hum instead.

Sometimes persistent throat clearing is a sign of having a dry throat (which itself may be a reaction to the same drugs that cause hoarseness). It may also be due to radiation therapy. More important, it can be a warning sign of throat cancer.

TREMBLY VOICE

If your voice is often shaky but you feel calm and collected, it may merely be a sign of aging. Or it can signal a neurological movement disorder called *essential tremor* of the head and neck, which is not usually terribly serious. The most common sign of essential tremor—also known as *familial tremor* because it tends to run in families—are hands that shake when trying to use them. But a shaky voice can also be a sign of more serious neurological disorders, such as *multiple sclerosis* and *Parkinson's disease*.

SLURRED SPEECH

Slurred speech at a cocktail party is likely to be a telltale sign of having had one too many. On the other hand, slurred speech—medically known as *dysarthria*—can signal a variety of medical conditions. For example, it can signal low blood sugar (*hypoglycemia*), a common complication of diabetes, as well as neurological disorders such as multiple sclerosis and Parkinson's disease. Unfortunately, because of their slurred speech, people with these serious conditions are often mistaken for being drunk.

In addition, slurred speech can be a dead giveaway that a person is having a mini-stroke—medically known as *transient ischemic attack* (*TIA*). It can also be a forewarning of a full-blown stroke. (See Appendix I.)

SIGN OF THE TIMES

During an interview in December 2006, South Dakota senator Tim Johnson groped for words and his speech became slurred. Johnson was displaying two of the classic signs of a stroke, confusion and difficulty communicating. He underwent surgery and was found to have a previously undetected birth defect, *arteriovenous malformation (AVM)*. AVM is an abnormal connection between an artery and a vein that—in Johnson's case—enlarged and burst.

STOP SIGN

Here are three simple steps a person should take to help tell if they are having a stroke:
1. Smile
2. Raise both arms
3. Repeat a simple sentence out loud like "The sky is blue"
If he or she has trouble with any of these tasks, call 911 immediately.

SUDDENLY SPEAKING WITH A FOREIGN ACCENT

If you wake up one morning and hear your partner speaking in a foreign accent, you might think you're still dreaming—or panic at the thought you went to bed with the wrong person. You may be relieved, at least at first, to discover that your bedmate probably has a very rare condition called *foreign accent* (or *language*) *syndrome*. While it sometimes signifies a psychological disorder, foreign accent syndrome is more likely a sign of brain damage, possibly from a head injury or stroke.

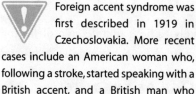

SIGNIFICANT FACT

Foreign accent syndrome was first described in 1919 in Czechoslovakia. More recent cases include an American woman who, following a stroke, started speaking with a British accent, and a British man who started speaking with an Italian accent after his stroke. A British woman, however, topped them both—she spoke with Slavic, French Canadian, and Jamaican accents following her stroke.

SPEAKING TOO LOUDLY OR TOO SOFTLY

Have you ever sat in a restaurant and one voice stood out loud and clear above the others? When someone speaks in an overly loud voice in public, in private, or on a cell phone, it can be extremely annoying. It may be a tip-off that the person is indeed annoying or seeking attention. But always speaking loudly is more often a sign of hearing loss. Conversely, a person who always speaks very softly, which can be just as annoying as speaking very loudly—there was even an entire episode of the TV series *Seinfeld* devoted to this subject—may also have hearing problems. Soft speakers may have what is known as *conductive hearing loss,* a condition in which a person hears his or her own voice (but not others' voices) amplified. Conductive hearing loss can be caused by the same factors that cause other types of hearing loss, including ear infections, growths, earwax, and blockage of the Eustachian tubes. (See Chapter 3.)

SIGNING OFF

As you can see, many throat, jaw, and neck signs are subtle, while others can be seen or heard loud and clear. In either case, don't hesitate to voice your concern if they trouble you. And any sudden sign—particularly those that are accompanied by bleeding, pain, or fever—should be checked out immediately.

To determine whether your sign points to something benign or serious, you can speak to your doctor or one of the following specialists:

- *Endocrinologist:* A medical doctor specially trained in diagnosing and treating diseases and disorders related to hormone production and imbalance.
- *Gastroenterologist:* A medical doctor who specializes in diagnosing and treating conditions of the digestive tract.
- *Otolaryngologist* (aka *otorhinolaryngologist*): A medical doctor who specializes in evaluating and treating ear, nose, and throat problems.
- *Pulmonologist:* A medical doctor who specializes in diseases and disorders of the lungs and respiratory system.
- *Speech Pathologists or Therapists:* Health care professionals who have advanced degrees in communication sciences. They provide speech rehabilitation to patients who have speech disorders or who have had strokes or brain injuries.

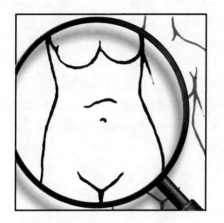

CHAPTER 7

THE MAIN BODY OF EVIDENCE

Your Torso and Extremities

The body says what words cannot.

—MARTHA GRAHAM, DANCER AND CHOREOGRAPHER

When we hear the word *body*, what's likely to spring to mind is the torso, not the head. Indeed, the mind is useless without the torso to carry out its wishes and whims. The body is the "temple of the soul," according to yoga philosophy. And both the 17th-century French philosopher Descartes and the 19th-century Russian writer Tolstoy viewed the body as a living machine.

The body, usually in the form of the naked torso, has been celebrated in art and literature throughout the ages. Michelangelo spent so much time studying and drawing Apollonios's sculpture *The Torso of Hercules* that he referred to himself as "the pupil of the torso." And there's an entire body of 16th-century French Renaissance poetry devoted to the body, called *blasons* and *contreblasons anatomiques*. The blazons (as they're spelled in English) celebrated the body, from the eyebrows to the "privy parts," while the counterblazons ridiculed them.

The Renaissance was an era when scientists, too, became obsessed with the human body. Despite Church laws forbidding them to do so, they began dissecting bodies whenever they could to understand better its workings. Though they learned that our heads house our brains and are the sole site of 4 out of 5 of our senses, they were much more fascinated with our torsos, the home to many of our most vital organs, including our hearts, lungs, intestines, kidneys, and liver, to name a few.

Luckily, today we don't usually have to dissect our bodies and pull out our organs to learn what's going on. If we stop, look, listen, touch, and smell, we can get all kinds of clues from our vital organs about things that may be going wrong inside. The shape and size of our bodies, our bodily sensations, the beating of our hearts, the way we stand and walk, and the look and feel of that mother of all body parts—our breasts—will reveal countless clues about our state of health.

BREASTS AND NIPPLES

MISMATCHED BREASTS

If you've ever looked closely at your breasts in a mirror, you've probably noticed that they're not mirror images of each other. One is often slightly larger, lower, or more off-center than the other. But if you find that one breast is a different cup size from its partner, it may be a sign of a usually benign—albeit cosmetically problematic—condition, appropriately called *breast asymmetry.* This discrepancy in breast size or shape can develop at any point but often first becomes apparent during puberty, when the breasts themselves are developing, or during pregnancy, when the breasts are preparing for breast-feeding.

WARNING SIGN

Women with asymmetrical breasts should be especially diligent about having mammograms. A recent British study found that even small irregularities in breast symmetry as measured by mammography may become an important indicator of increased risk of breast cancer.

Though rare, uneven breasts can also be a sign of a congenital defect called *Poland's syndrome*, in which the chest muscles on one side of the body are underdeveloped. Although present from birth, and sometimes hereditary, this type of breast asymmetry may go unnoticed until puberty when the breasts start to develop. Poland's syndrome is actually more common in men than women.

Sometimes other signs, such as webbed fingers (*syndactyly*) on the same side as the small breast, are noticeable. In general, Poland's syndrome doesn't usually cause serious problems. But some people with this condition do suffer from kidney and bladder problems. Last, but not least, mismatched breasts in both men and women are in important warning sign of breast cancer. (See **A Lump in the Breast**, below, and Appendix 1.)

SIGN OF THE TIMES

Amazon women—the women warriors of ancient Greek and other myths—were known not only for their fierce fighting prowess but for having only one breast. Indeed, the word *Amazon* is said to derive from the Greek *a mazos,* meaning "without breast." According to the legend, Amazon women cut or burned off their right breast to make it easier to shoot bows and arrows. These single-breasted warrior women—who some historians believe actually existed—are also credited with inventing the battle-axe. Unfortunately, the term *Amazon* has been used derogatorily against strong, powerful women.

A LUMP IN THE BREAST

If you've ever felt a lump in your breast, you've probably also felt your heart sink, your stomach drop, and your knees go weak. While a lump may indeed signal cancer, it's important to remember that 8 out of 10 breast lumps that are removed turn out not to be cancer. Breast lumps can be a sign of a number of benign conditions (as well as some not-so-benign ones).

It's not just women who get lumps in their breasts, and even breast cancer. Men do, too. While such cancers are rare, men between the ages of 60 and 70 are at the greatest risk. Interestingly, 20% of men with breast cancer have a close female relative who's had it.

LUMPY BREASTS

Many women notice lumpy breasts at certain times during their menstrual cycle as well as when they go through menopause. Some lumps in lumpy breasts can be precancerous. Usually, however, having lots of lumps (*diffuse lumpiness*) in the breast is more likely to signal a very common benign condition called *fibrocystic breast disease*—or, more accurately, *fibrocystic changes*. About 30% of women in the United States experience these breast changes. Although their exact cause is unknown, they are believed to be related to cyclical hormonal changes. Women with fibrocystic breasts often describe a feeling of breast heaviness or tenderness, particularly around the time of their periods. Some women describe their breasts as having a "cobblestone" feel. Sometimes women will also have nipple discharge. (See **Leaky Nipples,** below.) Fibrocystic breast disease, which can affect one or both breasts, tends to disappear after menopause.

If the skin around the lumps looks red or bruised, it may be a sign of *fat necrosis,* literally the death of fatty tissue. This sign is usually caused by a physical injury to the breast, which can cause fatty breast tissue to disintegrate. A woman—particularly if she's obese—may not even realize she's had a blow to her breast. However, some women may notice a nipple discharge on the breast that's been injured. (See **Leaky Nipples,** below.)

Lumpy breasts are hallmarks of two other common benign breast conditions, *cysts* (fluid-filled sacs) and *fibroadenomas* (solid masses). While breast cysts tend to occur in clusters, only one fibroadenoma is usually found as a solitary lump. Both types of lumps feel round, small, and firm, and both tend to move around under the skin when you press on them. (In fact, fibroadenomas can be so mobile that they've earned the unfortunate moniker **breast mice.**) Like the lumpiness of fibrocystic disease, these lumps tend to come and go in rhythm with a woman's menstrual cycle. Fibroadenomas are common even among teenage girls. They often become larger during pregnancy and lactation, and older women may notice more cysts during late menopause, if they're on hormone replacement therapy, or if they're very thin.

SWOLLEN, DISCOLORED BREASTS

While swollen breasts are a common sign that a woman is about to get her period, red *and* swollen breasts, particularly if they're warm to the touch, may be a sign of a very aggressive form of breast cancer, *inflammatory breast cancer (IBC)*. Pink, reddish purple, or bruised-looking breasts can also signal IBC.

Another classic sign of this deadly, fast-growing form of breast cancer is what doctors call *peau d'orange*—breast skin that has the kind of slightly dimpled surface and tiny indentations of an orange peel. Other IBC signs may include a feeling of breast heaviness or tenderness; burning, itching, or aching; change in the size or shape of the breast; and an inverted nipple. (See **Inverted Nipples,** below.) While many of these signs are also common during menstruation, IBC signs don't come and go. Rather, they tend to occur suddenly and increase steadily over weeks or months.

SIGNIFICANT FACT

The median age at time of diagnosis of breast cancer is 62. For inflammatory breast cancer it's 52.

IBC is often missed or misdiagnosed as an infection or even an insect bite because its signs are commonly seen on the surface of the breast. To confuse diagnostic matters further, the major sign of most breast cancers—a lump in the breast—is uncommon in women with IBC. (See **A Lump in the Breast,** above.)

WARNING SIGN

It's estimated that *inflammatory breast cancer (IBC)* accounts for 5 to 10% of breast cancer cases in the United States. In the 1990s, the incidence of IBC rose, as did survival rates. Both of these increases may be due to greater awareness and the use of mammograms.

Unlike more common forms of breast cancer, IBC tends to occur in younger women, particularly young African-American women. Inflammatory breast cancer rarely occurs in men, but when it does, it's usually found in older men.

ENLARGED BREASTS IN MEN

Large breasts in women are often seen as a sign of sexiness. Indeed, big-breasted women are likely to attract lots of attention, admiration, and even jealousy. But large breasts in men—medically known as *gynecomastia*—can attract ridicule. In gynecomastia, one or both breasts can be enlarged, and one can be even more enlarged than the other, resulting in breast asymmetry. (See **Mismatched Breasts,** above.) Men with gynecomastia often have another, less noticeable sign: a button- or disk-like lump under the nipple or around the areola.

SIGN OF THE TIMES

Male breast-feeding was recorded as far back as the Talmud, the ancient Jewish book of religion and law, and later in the Bible (Numbers 11–12).

More recently, in 1858, a German explorer described a Burmese peasant who nursed his baby for five months after his wife fell ill.

Scottish missionary David Livingstone (of "I presume" fame) also reported observing men breast-feeding their infants.

In 2002, a Sri Lankan man whose wife died in childbirth breast-fed his 2 infant daughters for more than 3 months.

This condition is especially common among obese men. Astonishingly, 70% of boys will experience a mild form of gynecomastia during puberty. In these cases, the enlarged breasts are usually benign signs of the natural hormonal fluctuations of puberty. Hormone-related gynecomastia is also seen in older men and is a sign of what's been medically dubbed *andropause,* the male equivalent of menopause. Just as women lose estrogen as they age and go through menopause, men lose androgen.

About 1 in 4 adult men with enlarged breasts appear to have no underlying medical problem. However, in the remainder, a medical cause can be found. For example, gynecomastia is a revealing sign of a rare genetic condition called *Klinefelter's syndrome,* which is a leading cause of male sterility (see Chapter 1) and raises the risk of breast cancer in men. Enlarged breasts in men can also be a warning sign of a pituitary tumor, a liver disorder, or even testicular cancer. Gynecomastia can also be a reaction to any one of a myriad of medicines commonly prescribed to men, including those to treat baldness, ulcers, heartburn, high blood pressure, depression, heart failure, or prostate problems. Or it can signal marijuana or steroid use and abuse.

WARNING SIGN

Because men with Klinefelter's syndrome have higher-than-normal estrogen levels, they're at increased risk of breast cancer. If you have this disorder be on the lookout for signs of breast cancer, such as swollen breasts and nipple discharge.

Finally, breast swelling in men, as in women, may signal certain benign breast disorders such as *papillomas* and *fibroadenomas* (noncancerous growths in the milk ducts) (see **Lumpy Breasts,** above), but it can also be a warning sign of breast cancer.

WARNING SIGN

Because the liver plays a critical role in hormone metabolism, men with liver disorders are at increased risk of developing *gynecomastia* and breast cancer.

EXTRA BREASTS

Many of us have marveled at the sight of a pack of pups suckling at their mother's teats. And we might have seen pictures and statues of fertility goddesses with rows of breasts across their chests. Perhaps we've thought that multiple breasts in humans were just the stuff of fantasies. But some people do have one or more extra breasts—medically called *polymastia*. Also known as *supernumerary breasts,* they can come with or without nipples and areolae. (See **Triple Nipples,** below.) Most often these mammary marvels are not noticed until puberty, when they start to develop in response to sex hormones.

SIGN OF THE TIMES

Anne Boleyn, the second wife of Henry VIII, was said to have a third breast—to say nothing of a goiter and an extra finger. If true, it might explain why a Venetian ambassador was claimed to have said that she "was not one of the handsomest women in the world."

Extra breasts don't just arise on the chest; they can develop on the buttocks, neck, shoulders, and back as well. And both men and women can have them. While multiple breasts can certainly be a cosmetic concern, any problem that can develop in a normal breast—including cancer—can occur in an extra one as well. And defects in the kidneys and other organs are sometimes seen in people with extra breasts.

TRIPLE NIPPLES

Two's company, three's a . . . well, a weird sign when it comes to nipples. Triple nipples—medically called *supernumerary nipples* or *polythelia*—are often a very subtle birth anomaly. These nonfunctioning (vestigial), superfluous nipples are sometimes described as slightly deformed miniatures of the real thing. The extra nipple is usually found on the chest or the lower abdomen along what's known as the "milk line"—that is, where nipples are usually located in other mammals. They can also pop up on the neck, armpit, or just about anywhere else on the body. Some even occur on the forehead, where they may look like little freckles or pimples. Occasionally the extra nipples—and tissue beneath them—develop into full-blown breasts when awash in sex hormones during puberty or pregnancy. There have even been reports of extra nipples, as well as extra breasts, producing milk.

SIGNIFICANT FACT

If you want to know if your odd bump is a freckle or a triple nipple, place an ice cube on it. If it pops out, it's a nipple.

SIGN OF THE TIMES

In medieval England, triple nipples were considered a witches' mark. Demons and other unworldly creatures were thought to suckle from the extra nipples.

Triple, quadruple, or even more nipples are not that unusual. Indeed, an estimated 5% of children are born with them. They seem to be more common, however, among Native American women.

While usually benign, multiple nipples may be a sign of a myriad of medical conditions—from skeletal deformities to ulcers, from migraines to gallbladder problems. And like extra breasts, extra nipples can be a sign of rare genetic kidney and urinary tract defects. These defects are more likely to be seen in men with super-numerary nipples than in women with them.

INVERTED NIPPLES

We all expect our nipples to look like . . . well, nipples—pointed and perky. But sometimes our nipples look more like dimples. Medically known as *inverted nipples,* they can be a benign sign or signal something more serious.

Women and men who are born with "innie" rather than "outie" nipples usually have nothing to worry about—although women may be embarrassed about having inverted nipples, and they may find breast-feeding difficult. However, if a normally pointy nipple changes and becomes inverted, this may be a warning sign of breast cancer, especially if there's also a bloody discharge or lump near the nipple. (See **Leaky Nipples,** below, and **A Lump in the Breast,** above.)

HEALTHY SIGN

Bluish veins visible on the breast are a healthy sign of pregnancy. In fact, they're one of the earliest. They signal the breast is getting ready to produce milk.

CRUSTY NIPPLES

Nipples and the areola surrounding them should be soft and supple. But if you notice some crusty or scaly skin, it can be a sign of *Paget's disease of the breast* (sometimes called *Paget's disease of the nipple*), a type of breast cancer. The crusty skin actually contains cancer cells. Found primarily in women, Paget's disease of the breast is a medical condition that shouldn't be confused with another disease called *Paget's disease,* which is a bone disorder.

WARNING SIGN

A nipple that looks like it has eczema should not be ignored. Unfortunately, 9 out of 10 women who have this sign have breast cancer.

Typically, only one nipple is affected in Paget's disease of the breast. The nipple may be flattened or inverted and may produce a straw-colored or bright red discharge. (See **Non-Milky Discharge,** below.) Other signs include flaky skin, redness, itching, and burning, much like signs of the skin condition eczema. These signs may come and go, making a woman—and sometimes her doctor—think that she has just a simple recurrent skin condition. Unfortunately, many women with Paget's disease of the breast have these warning signs for 6 or 8 months before their cancer is diagnosed. This may be because they put off going to their doctor, or their doctor initially attributed the signs to another disorder.

As with other forms of breast cancer, Paget's disease of the breast can be classified two ways: either as *ductal carcinoma in situ (DCIS),* which is a very early stage of breast cancer with cancer cells that are confined to the milk ducts, or as *invasive ductal carcinoma,* a late-stage with cancer that has spread from the ducts into the surrounding breast tissue.

SIGNIFICANT FACTS

Besides a breast lump, here are other signs of breast cancer:

- Crusty or scaly nipples
- Inverted nipples
- Bloody nipple discharge
- Redness or swelling of the breast
- Breast skin that resembles the texture of an orange peel (peau d'orange)
- Breast asymmetry
- A sore or ulcer that doesn't heal

LEAKY NIPPLES

If you've ever breast-fed, you know full well that leaky breasts are a telltale sign that your baby needs to nurse or that you need to pump milk right away. While leaky nipples in a new mother are a healthy sign of lactation, nipple discharge in others can be alarming at best and a sign of some serious conditions at worst. The type of nipple discharge, whether it's coming from one or both breasts, and from where on

SIGN OF THE TIMES

Although it is rare, some women who've had their nipples pierced have experienced milk production and leakage.

the nipple it's sprouting are all clues to the sign's significance. Medically, leaks from a nipple are classified as either milky or non-milky. While a milky leak is clearly milky-looking, a non-milky leak can be clear, yellow, straw-like, green, brown, pink, or bright red. Complicating matters, different types of discharge may occur in some breast disorders. In general, nipple discharge is considered to be *pathologic* (caused by a disease) if it occurs on its own, only comes from one milk duct, happens repeatedly, or is bloody.

SIGNIFICANT FACT

Of the women who have an abnormal nipple discharge, less than 10% actually have breast cancer. The older a woman is, however, the more likely it is that nipple discharge will be her only sign of breast cancer.

Milky Discharge

A milky nipple discharge in a woman who's not pregnant or nursing, or in a man, is medically known as *galactorrhea*. Usually this occurs in both breasts, and the discharge is thin and whitish, or possibly milky yellow or green. While in adults it's usually a sign of a medical condition, during puberty both girls and boys may have a benign milky discharge. Interestingly, about 5% of newborn babies will leak milk from their breasts.

SIGNIFICANT FACT

Women who adopt can breastfeed their babies. By stimulating their breasts for several weeks with a manual or mechanical pump—a technique known as *induced lactation*—they can often produce small quantities of milk. If so, they and their babies can reap the emotional and health benefits of breastfeeding.

Usually galactorrhea is seen in both breasts, and the discharge is thin and whitish. Breasts can leak after vigorous rubbing, squeezing, or sucking, in which case it's a benign sign.

WARNING SIGN

In men, a milky discharge is often the only sign of breast cancer. In women, however, having milky discharge without other signs is less likely to signal a serious problem.

Galactorrhea can be a reaction to both prescription and illicit drugs, including birth control pills, hormone replacement therapy, antipsychotics, antidepressants, antihypertensives, marijuana, opiates, and steroids. A milky discharge can also be a sign you've been eating a lot of phytoestrogen-containing herbs, such as nettle, fennel, blessed thistle, anise, and fenugreek seed. The estrogen in these herbs can cause milk to flow. Leaking milk can also signal several hormone-related conditions, including a pituitary tumor (*prolactinoma*) and *hypothyroidism*. (See Appendix I.)

Non-Milky Discharge

A greenish or dark, thick, sticky nipple discharge may signal clogged and inflamed milk ducts, a benign but unpleasant condition called *mammary duct ectasia*. The discharge can come from one or more of the tiny ducts that lead to the nipple. But a pus-like, foul-smelling discharge may signal a breast infection—medically known as *mastitis*. And a bright red, blood-like discharge from only one milk duct on the nipple is a classic sign of the noncancerous growth called *intraductal papilloma*.

A reddish discharge, particularly from only one milk duct, may be a red flag for two forms of breast cancer—Paget's disease of the breast and ductal carcinoma in situ. (See **Crusty Nipples,** above.)

Finally, whether bloody or not, nipple discharge from several milk ducts is a common sign of fibrocystic changes (see **Lumpy Breasts,** above) or other benign breast conditions.

Spontaneous discharge from one duct—which may or may not look bloody—is the hallmark of an *intraductal papilloma,* a noncancerous

SIGNIFICANT FACT

The only way to determine if a breast change is benign or more serious is what's medically known as "the triple test":

- A clinical breast examination, which is one done by a health care professional
- Imaging—a mammogram or ultrasound
- A nonsurgical biopsy—a fine-needle aspiration and/or core biopsy

If any one of the results is positive, then further evaluation is needed. And remember, not just lumps need to be checked out. So do any leaks or changes in shape, size, skin, or sensation.

growth in a milk duct. Although usually not noticeable, some women do describe seeing a small wart-like bump behind or near the edge of the nipple. Such bumps may appear on one or both breasts. Interestingly, younger women tend to have multiple growths, while older women usually have only one.

BODY SHAPE AND SIZE

APPLE-SHAPED BODY

An apple a day may keep the doctor away, but if you're shaped like an apple, with extra weight around the midsection, you'll want to keep your doctor around. This body type is medically known as *central* or *visceral adiposity* or popularly as beer- or potbelly. Belly fat actually releases dangerous fatty acids that build up in the liver. This can hamper the body's metabolization of sugar and raise the risk of diabetes.

Having a fatty middle can signal *metabolic syndrome,* a cluster of diabetes and heart disease risk factors that includes insulin resistance, high blood pressure, high blood sugar, high triglyceride levels, and low HDL (high-density lipoprotein or "good" cholesterol) levels. Indeed, people who are apple-shaped are three times more likely to suffer a heart attack than those who are pear-shaped—that is, carrying most of their fat in their buttocks.

WARNING SIGN

High triglycerides and low HDL levels are stronger risk factors for heart disease in women than in men.

An apple-shaped body is a serious sign that you're also at increased risk for colon cancer. In fact, belly fat is such an important predictor of heart and other diseases that measuring waist circumference during a physical examination may soon become as commonplace as taking your height and weight—and much more revealing. Studies are now showing that waist circumference alone is a better predictor of future cardiovascular problems than just weight or other measures, such as body mass index (BMI) or waist-hip ratio (WHR).

WARNING SIGNS

A 40-inch waistline in men and a 35-inch waist in women places them at increased risk of heart disease. And women with a 36-inch or larger waist are at increased risk of gallstones.

Unfortunately, many menopausal women find that as their age creeps up, so does their weight. Besides being distressing, a gain of more than 44 pounds after menopause puts a woman at increased risk of breast cancer. And the extra pounds can be a forewarning of looming heart trouble. However, it's unclear whether putting on weight later in life is more harmful for women than being overweight for many years.

SUDDEN OR UNEXPLAINED WEIGHT CHANGE

Seeing the numbers on our bathroom scales dipping can be a welcome sign of success in our battle against the bulge. But any sudden and unintended shift in weight—in either direction—is a sure sign that something is seriously wrong.

Of course, rapid, self-induced weight loss can signal an eating disorder, such as *anorexia* or *bulimia*. But unintended weight loss, with or without loss of appetite, can point to depression, diabetes, hyperthyroidism, heart failure, a nutritional disorder, or cancer. A recent study found that unexplained weight loss in women may be an early warning sign of dementia a decade later. And sudden weight loss can be a reaction to some drugs—both prescribed and illicit—including antidepressants and amphetamines. If an older adult loses weight suddenly, it may be a forewarning of dementia. While it's common for the elderly to lose weight as they age—usually less than a pound a year—losing more than that appears to signal the imminent onset of this neurological disorder.

We've probably all experienced putting on a few extra pounds, especially around the holidays. This is usually a benign sign of lack of restraint around the buffet table. But sudden weight gain can also signal some serious and not-so-serious systemic problems.

Putting on weight in a matter of a day or two can be due to fluid retention (*edema*). Many women notice that both their breasts and bellies bloat as they retain water just before their periods. But fluid retention can also signal *heart failure*, the inability of the heart to pump efficiently. Although swollen feet and legs are classic signs of heart failure, heart-disease-related edema can build up around the abdomen as well.

If you've been putting on pounds and then dropping them dramatically without changing your eating habits, it may signal a number of physical or psychological problems. Up-and-down weight gain and loss can, for example, be a clue that you have a thyroid disorder (see Appendix I), an infection, a nutritional problem, or an eating disorder.

SIGN OF THE TIMES

 In the 1940s, an American psychologist, William Sheldon, identified three basic body types, which he called *somatotypes,* and linked them to personality traits.

- *Ectomorph:* Thin, delicate body. Tends to be nonassertive, sensitive, self-conscious, introverted, and artistic.
- *Endomorph:* Plump, apple- or pear-shaped body. Tends to be sluggish, even-tempered, affectionate, sociable, and "a barrel of fun."
- *Mesomorph:* Muscular and athletic. Tends to be active, adventuresome, risk-taking, competitive, assertive, and indifferent to others.

WARNING SIGN

 "Yo-yo" weight gain and loss isn't just frustrating. In men, it can be a sign that they're at increased risk of developing gallstones. The large Health Professionals Follow-up Study found that repeated weight loss and gain in men, particularly if they lost more than 20 pounds in a dieting episode, might increase their risk of gallstones by 50%.

SHRINKING

The Incredible Shrinking Man entertained millions of moviegoers. But if you're the one who's shrinking, you're not likely to be amused. Losing height is a fairly common sign of aging. But, according to a recent British study, older men who lose more than one inch are at increased risk of death from heart and respiratory conditions.

Losing height is also a hallmark of osteoporosis, a serious disease that involves the loss of bone in both men and women. (See **Hunched Back,** below.) Women, however, are 4 times more likely than men to develop it because of menopause-related loss of bone mass. Because of the bone loss in osteoporosis, the spine can sustain tiny fractures, called *vertebral compression fractures.* Over time, the spinal structures pancake on themselves, resulting in a noticeable loss of height.

CURVED BACK

A crooked back can signal *scoliosis,* a curvature of the spine. The curve is almost always noticed first by others and can be seen most easily when you bend over from the waist. Sometimes people with scoliosis will spy the problem themselves; for example, they may notice that one shoulder or one hip is higher than the other when they look at themselves in a mirror. While many people first develop it in childhood, this spinal deformity can begin, or can worsen and become more noticeable, in adulthood. Adult-onset scoliosis is another body sign of aging and is largely due to wear and tear on the structures that support the spine. Or it may be due to a degenerative joint condition. Whatever the cause, scoliosis can lead to difficulty walking and pain.

HUNCHED BACK

Have you ever noticed that many old people, especially women, walk hunched over and have a large rounded hump on their upper back? This deformity is commonly called a "dowager's hump" or "widow's hump"—

medically known as *kyphosis.* Unlike people with scoliosis, who look like they're tilting to the side, those with kyphosis look like they're bending forward.

Kyphosis is a classic sign of *osteoporosis.* (See **Shrinking,** above.) Unfortunately, osteoporosis has no early warning signs; its first indication may be the dowager hump, or a broken bone or hip. The hump can also be a telltale sign of tuberculosis, a spinal tumor or injury, or degenerative arthritis. (See **Stiff Joints,** below.)

SPEAKING OF SIGNS

The spine is a series of bones running down your back. You sit on one end of it and your head sits on the other.

—Anonymous

WARNING SIGN

An osteoporosis-related hip fracture is a warning sign of increased risk of death. Nearly 1 out of 4 people older than 50 who break a hip die in the year following the fracture. Many of those who survive will require long-term care because they're left with significant trouble walking.

UNGAINLY GAIT

UNSTEADINESS

If your elderly aunt seems unsteady on her feet, or tends to lean backward when standing or even sitting, it may be a sign of a newly recognized posture disorder named *psychomotor disadaptation syndrome (PDS).* Hesitating when starting to walk and a tendency to take small steps with a shuffling gait—medically called *marche à petits pas*—are characteristics of this condition. A fear of falling is also another characteristic sign of this disorder. PDS is sometimes mistaken for Parkinson's disease and other neuromuscular disorders. (See **Tremors,** below.)

SIGNIFICANT FACT

Researchers believe that inactivity may actually worsen or increase the risk of PDS. Being confined to bed for an illness can trigger it in older folks, too. This is confirmation of the use-it-or-lose-it approach to health.

Besides being a common sign of aging, PDS may point to a number of serious conditions, such as heart disease, dehydration, and low blood sugar (*hypoglycemia*) or other metabolic problems. PDS can also signal changes in the small blood vessels in the brain or even a brain tumor.

STIFF, RIGID GAIT

If you've ever seen a person who walks ramrod straight, like a tin soldier, he or she is probably suffering from *stiff-man syndrome*. This rare neurological disorder is also known as *stiff-person syndrome* (**SPS**), which is not only more politically correct but also more accurate, because the condition affects both men and women.

SPS causes recurring bouts of muscle stiffness and spasms and is thought to be an autoimmune disorder. Indeed, it's more prevalent among people who have other autoimmune diseases, such as pernicious anemia, insulin-dependent diabetes, and hyperthyroidism. (See Appendix I.)

The signs of stiff-person syndrome usually appear first in the muscles of the trunk. As it progresses, it spreads to the limbs and may cause joint deformity, other joint and skeletal problems, and disability.

Attacks are often set off when the person is emotionally stressed or something, such as a loud noise, suddenly scares or surprises the person. Unfortunately, stiff-person syndrome is often misdiagnosed as a psychological disorder, multiple sclerosis, or Parkinson's disease, thus delaying appropriate treatment.

JOINTS

DOUBLE-JOINTEDNESS

Have you ever seen people bend their fingers all the way back or even twist their whole bodies like a human pretzel? They may be displaying the classic signs of *hypermobility syndrome*, aka *hyperflexibility* or **double-jointedness**. People with this condition don't really have a double set of joints; rather the ligaments and muscles around their joints are superflexible, resulting in the ability to bend and stretch like a contortionist. This is generally a benign condition that usually becomes evident in childhood and tends to run in families. Up to 20% of normal children have hyper-flexible joints, as do many athletes. However, some people develop hyper-mobility in later life if their ligaments become injured, weakened, or overly stretched. Regardless of when or how it occurs, people with hypermobile joints may be at in-creased risk for joint dislocations and pain.

It's long been believed that hy-perflexible joints are harbingers of *osteoarthritis*, a degenerative joint disorder. (See **Stiff Joints**, below.) But this hasn't been proven, at least

SIGN OF THE TIMES

Hypermobility can come in handy for musicians as well as athletes. The 19th-century Italian violinist Paganini and the 20th-century Russian pianist Rachmaninoff are said to have had this condition, which worked to their advantage. It's believed that their long, flexible limbs were the re-sult of Marfan syndrome.

as far as the hands and fingers go. In fact, being double-jointed might pro-tect against arthritis, according to a recent study. On the other hand, hav-ing hyperflexible joints may be a forewarning of *chronic fatigue syndrome,* a condition thought to be caused by a virus and characterized by excessive fatigue, weakness, muscle pain, and sometimes fever. A higher incidence of hyperflexible joints has been seen in both young peo-ple and adults with chronic fatigue syndrome.

Two potentially serious but often undiagnosed genetic conditions that are frequently associated with joint hypermobility are *Ehlers-Danlos syn-drome* and *Marfan syndrome.* Ehlers-Danlos syndrome (EDS) is a rare connective tissue disorder primarily affecting the joints, skin, and blood vessels. Other EDS signs, which range from mild to severe, may include very stretchable (lax) skin (see Chapter 9), easy bruising, joint dislocation, *scoliosis* (see **Curved Back,** above), eye problems, and ruptured arteries, bowel, or other organs. EDS is potentially debilitating and even life-threatening. But because the signs of EDS can be so subtle, it goes un-diagnosed in an estimated 90% of people with the disorder until they seek attention for a medical emergency.

Hypermobile joints are also a sign of Marfan syndrome, another rare connective tissue disorder. Other visible signs of Marfan may include flat long feet, a narrow face, scoliosis, long, thin fingers, and tall stature.

(Abraham Lincoln had long, thin fingers and is said to have had this condition.) Although Marfan's primarily affects the skeleton, it can cause eye, cardiac, and other problems as well. Indeed, many people with this condition are very nearsighted and/or have glaucoma or cataracts.

As with EDS, the subtle signs of Marfan's are often overlooked, sometimes with disastrous consequences. Many young athletes, for example, have hyperflexible joints and are tall with long extremities—characteristics that help in sports. But some may have undiagnosed Marfan's. Sad to say, a number of these young athletes die suddenly and unnecessarily each year because they were unaware they had this condition. Aortic aneurysm—a ballooning and possible rupture of the body's largest blood vessel—is a major cause of early death in untreated Marfan's.

STIFF JOINTS

While some people have extremely flexible joints, other people's joints are so stiff it's as though they're frozen. But having stiff joints can be a benign sign that you've overindulged in your favorite sport. Or it may signal the opposite—you haven't been active enough. Unfortunately, stiffness may discourage people from being more physically active, which in turn can worsen the stiffness. If joint stiffness is accompanied by persistent joint pain, you can be pretty sure something is wrong.

If you're past middle age, stiff joints are most likely yet another annoying, but usually benign, sign of aging. What keeps your joints capable of moving through a full range of motion with ease and comfort is *synovial fluid,* which is secreted by the membranes surrounding the joints.

With aging, there's less of this lubrication, and moving the joints becomes more difficult. Joint stiffness, regardless of your age, is often worse in the morning or after being inactive for long periods of time, as when sitting in a theater or on a plane. As you move about during the day, the stiffness usually dissipates.

While chronic morning stiffness can be a sign that you need a new mattress, it's also a common sign of arthritis. In fact,

SPEAKING OF SIGNS

A woman is as young as her knees.
—Mary Quant, British fashion designer

morning stiffness is its hallmark. If the morning stiffness lasts for less than 30 minutes, it's likely a sign of osteoarthritis (OA). Often called the "wear-and-tear" form of arthritis, OA—also known as *degenerative arthritis*—is the most common form of the more than 100 different types of arthritis. OA destroys the cushioning cartilage between the joints, which eventually causes bone to rub up against bone, leading to pain, deformity, and loss of function. While OA can involve any joint in the body, the hips, knees, feet, and fingers are most often affected. It occurs more often in men than women before the age of 45 but is more common in women over the age of 55.

WARNING SIGN

If a painless joint hurts when you apply pressure on it, you may have osteoarthritis.

If morning stiffness lasts longer than 30 minutes, it's more likely to be *rheumatoid arthritis (RA),* a progressive, debilitating immune disease that can affect not only the joints but other parts of the body, including the tear ducts and salivary glands, as well.

Stiff joints any time of day can signal a number of muscular, skeletal, or neurological conditions. These can include the inflammatory conditions *lupus* (see Appendix I); and *sarcoidosis* (see **Body Tingling and Numbness**, below, and Appendix I); as well as the muscular condition *fibromyalgia* (see **Cold Hands and Feet**, below).

Joint stiffness can also be a reaction to a number of drugs, including antibiotics such as minocycline, statins (used to lower cholesterol), and aromatase inhibitors (used to treat breast cancer).

WARNING SIGN

People with rheumatoid arthritis are at increased risk of suffering a heart attack or stroke.

CREAKY KNEES

Do your knees make you sound like the Tin Man from *The Wizard of Oz*? If there's no pain involved, your creaky knees may be a sign of some benign temporary mechanical maladjustment. For example, the soft tissue in the joint (the patella) is slightly misaligned and rubbing up against nearby tissue. Or it may be that these elastic-like soft tissues, such as the tendons and ligaments, are snapping back around the knees after momentarily sliding out of place. Or, similar to what happens when cracking the knuckles, tiny gas bubbles normally found in the synovial fluid that lubricates the joints, pop out.

But noisy knees can also signal the onset of OA of the knee. (See **Stiff Joints,** above.) Knee OA and other knee problems are more prevalent in women than men and tend to increase around menopause. There's some evidence that the drop in estrogen is to blame.

SIGNIFICANT FACTS

Here are some other differences between *osteoarthritis (OA)* and *rheumatoid arthritis (RA)*:

- RA usually affects joints symmetrically. For example, both hands or both knees are likely to be affected. OA usually affects only one side at a time.
- RA can cause fatigue and low-grade fever. OA doesn't.
- OA causes joint and muscle pain that worsens as the day's activities go on. RA tends to be equally bad throughout the day.

HAND AND FOOT SIGNS

BEING LEFT-HANDED

If you're left-handed, you probably realize you're in the minority. In fact, only about 10% of the population are "southpaws" or "lefties," as left-handed people are sometimes called. This trait is thought to be primarily genetic (inherited) or congenital (present at birth). In the latter case, it's hypothesized the left-handedness is the result of exposure to abnormally high levels of testosterone in the womb.

Left-handedness can be not just an inconvenience but a marker for a number of autoimmune disorders, especially thyroid disease (see Appendix I) and *inflammatory bowel disease (IBD)*, which encompasses *Crohn's disease* and *ulcerative colitis*. (See Chapter 8.) In addition, being left-handed has been linked to some behavioral problems. Some of these problems, however, may be partly the result of parents or teachers trying to force lefties into being righties, a practice that is still widespread in some parts of the world.

A recent Dutch study found preliminary evidence that left-handed women were at increased risk for developing premenopausal breast cancer. But the news isn't all bad for southpaws. Lefties appear

SIGNIFICANT FACT

Several surveys indicate that there is more left-handedness in the young than in the old. Some researchers contend that this is the result of social pressure to become right-handed. Other, more skeptical—or, some might say, sinister—scientists claim that the dearth of left-handed elders means that left-handedness predisposes humans to an early death.

SIGN OF THE TIMES

Among famous southpaws are Leonardo da Vinci, President George H. W. Bush, President Bill Clinton, and Oprah Winfrey.

SIGN OF THE TIMES

Left-handed people used to be considered evil. Indeed, the word *sinister* is derived from the Latin *sinistra,* which means "left." In more recent times, lefties were sometimes even accused of being "leftists," that is, communists.

to have better memories than righties, as well as an advantage in hand-to-hand combat. And according to a French study, they tend to excel at such sports as baseball, tennis, and fencing.

KNOBBY KNUCKLES

As children, many of us were scared by images of mean old ladies with gnarled hands going after small children. (Think the witch in the story of Hansel and Gretel.) Most women with knobby knuckles, however, are displaying the mark of *hand osteoarthritis,* not of meanness. These painful bone growths on the fingers are unfortunate signs of aging that are especially common in older women. They're sometimes medically called *Heberden's node* or *Bouchard's node*, depending on which finger and which joint is affected.

WARNING SIGN

It's long been believed that frequently cracking your knuckles can lead to arthritis. There is, however, no evidence to support this theory. On the other hand, frequent knuckle popping can cause soft-tissue damage in the joints, as well as a decrease in the hand's gripping ability.

CLUB-LIKE FINGERS

If someone's misshapen fingers look more like drumsticks than a witch's hand, that person may have what's known as *clubbed fingers*. (See Chapter 9.) The clubbing can strike one or both hands, and sometimes only one finger.

SIGN OF THE TIMES

Clubbed fingers are considered the oldest clinical sign in medicine. Hippocrates was the first to describe clubbing in patients with lung disease. To this day, this sign is sometimes referred to as *Hippocratic fingers*.

Clubbed fingers—digital clubbing, as the condition is also called—usually develop very gradually and painlessly. Unfortunately, they can be a sign of several serious conditions, especially if there are nail changes as well. About one in three people with lung cancer have this sign. Clubbed fingers can also signal other cancers and such lung diseases as *cystic fibrosis* and *tuberculosis*. In addition, they can be markers for Crohn's disease and ulcerative colitis (see Chapter 8), and for heart disease, hyperthyroidism (see Appendix I), and liver disease.

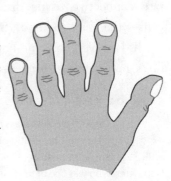

CLUBBED FINGERS

CURLED FINGERS

Have you ever noticed someone whose fingers are always bent like a claw? If so, that person is displaying the classic sign of *Dupuytren's disease (DD)* or *Dupuytren's contracture,* a rare, slowly progressing, and painless but debilitating disorder. This condition often starts with a small nodule in the palm and then progresses to a thickening and scarring of the connective tissue in the palm and fingers. As a result, the fingers—

SIGN OF THE TIMES

Dupuytren's disease is thought to have originated with the Vikings, who conquered the British Isles and much of northern Europe. Through intermarriage, they spread the disease throughout these areas.

usually the ring finger and pinky—permanently curl, the hallmark of this condition.

Although the cause is unknown, some people may have a genetic predisposition. DD is most prevalent among whites of northern European (especially Scandinavian) descent and is more common in men than women. Smokers and heavy drinkers are at increased risk. One or both hands may be affected. The ring finger is affected most often, followed by the little, middle, and index fingers.

Dupuytren's is often seen in people with diabetes; in fact, it's been estimated to occur in up to two-thirds of people who've had diabetes for many years. It can also be a clue that a person is suffering from epilepsy or a thyroid, liver, or lung disease. People with DD may also have other rare connective tissue disorders, including *Peyronie's disease*, which causes the penis to bend. (See Chapter 8.)

If, however, only one finger is locked in a curled position, it's a sure-fire sign of a *trigger finger*—medically known as ***stenosing tenosynovitis.*** This condition tends to affect people who engage in repetitive hand and finger movements at work or play, such as at a computer keyboard. People who spend a lot of time gripping hard objects, such as power tools, garden tools, or even musical instruments, are also at increased risk for this condition. These strenuous activities trigger tiny injuries to the fingers. Also at risk are people with diabetes, hypothyroidism, rheumatoid arthritis, and some lung and skin infections. Women are more likely than men to suffer from trigger finger.

Although some people with Dupuytren's disease also have trigger finger, the conditions are medically different. Moreover, trigger finger can cause more pain than Dupuytren's. People with trigger finger usually have more stiffness and discomfort in the morning.

BUMP ON THE WRIST OR HAND

Finding a lump anywhere can be pretty frightening. But if you've recently developed one on your hand or the back of your wrist, you probably have nothing to wring your hands over. It's most likely a sign of ***ganglion cyst,*** a benign fluid-filled lump. These cysts can actually pop up anywhere—on the hand and fingers and on other parts of the body as well. Women are more likely to have them than men, and they're especially common in gymnasts.

The bump swells with physical activity and decreases when the hand is at rest. Although they can be tender and achy, ganglion cysts tend to be more unsightly than painful. The good news is that even if untreated, almost one-third of these cysts will disappear on their own.

A lump on the hand can also be a sign of gout or rheumatoid arthritis. But people with these conditions are likely to have pain and other signs.

TWISTED TOES

If the toes between your big toe and your pinky toe look like inverted V's—or more like a hawk's foot than a human's—it's likely the telltale sign of *hammertoe,* a common foot deformity. With hammertoe, the toe is bent at the middle joint. Indeed, as its name suggests, the toes buckle and point downward, giving the toe a hammer-like look.

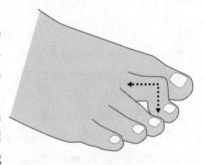

Hammertoes are usually a benign but unattractive and sometimes painful sign that you're wearing the wrong shoes. If your shoes don't allow your toes to stretch out when you walk, your toes can bend permanently.

HAMMERTOE

If you find yourself buying wider and wider shoes and your big toe is pointing out to the side rather than straight ahead, you have the classic sign of a *bunion.* While bony protrusions at the base of the big toe are the hallmarks of a bunion, a similar protrusion at the base of the little toe is called a *bunionette.* A bunion—medically known as *hallux valgus*—can get quite large and cause the big toe to crunch into or grow under its neighbor. Swelling and redness are other common

SIGN OF THE TIMES

Famed anthropologist Margaret Mead observed that many members of a South Seas island tribe had bunions, yet they had never worn shoes! A bunion is usually the result of inherited faulty foot mechanics, which put abnormal stress on the front of the foot.

signs of bunions, which can produce mild to severe pain.

Bunions tend to be more common in families and in people with flat feet or low arches. There's some controversy about the real cause of bunions. Some believe that, as with hammertoes, they're proof positive that you've been trying to cram your feet into shoes that are too small, too narrow, or too high-heeled. Others insist that bunions are due to an inherited mechanical imbalance that puts undue stress on the big toe. Most agree that both are factors. Bunions can also be an early warning sign that arthritis is just a step or two behind.

SIGNIFICANT FACT

Half the women in America have bunions.

A BUMP ON YOUR HEEL

If you're having difficulty getting those slingbacks on because of a bone growing on the back of your heel, you may have *posterior calcaneal exostosis,* aka "pump bumps." This bony protrusion, which also goes by the name *Haglund's deformity,* is characterized by enlargement of the large bone of the heel (*calcaneus*).

These pump bumps can be painful, particularly if you develop *bursitis*—an inflammation of the small fluid-filled sacs (*bursa*) that lubricate and cushion joints throughout the body—from repeatedly wearing shoes that put pressure on the backs of your feet. But they can be hereditary as well.

WEIRD BODY SENSATIONS AND MOVEMENTS

BODY TINGLING AND NUMBNESS

Feeling tingly all over may sound pleasurable, and it can be. A warm bath, an invigorating massage, and sex can all give us a tingly feeling. But having a tingling tush—medically known as *buttock paresthesia*—may be a sign of something more than a sensuous lifestyle. Paresthesias are abnormal sensations, such as tingling, numbness, burning, prickling, a pins-and-needles feeling, or the sensation that a foot or arm has fallen asleep.

Buttock paresthesia may signal a *pinched nerve*—as can paresthesia on any part of the body. Pinched nerves can be caused by repetitive movements, joint and spinal injuries or diseases, and even pregnancy. A very common form of chronically pinched nerves is known as *nerve entrapment syndrome*. Entrapment disorders include *tennis elbow; carpal tunnel syndrome,* which affects the hands, wrists, and forearms (see **Tingly, Numb Fingers,** below); and *tarsal tunnel syndrome,* which affects the feet (see **Tingly, Numb Feet,** below).

Paresthesia can also be a sign of many other conditions that may or may not be related to pinched nerves. These include pregnancy, spinal injuries or conditions such as ruptured or herniated discs, and brain abscesses or tumors.

Occasionally, numbness and tingling are forewarnings (aka *auras*) of a migraine or epileptic seizure. They may also signal *sensory seizures,* a type of epilepsy involving distortions of the senses rather than convulsions. And feeling numb and tingly can be a sign of several serious systemic and autoimmune conditions including hypothyroidism, diabetes, and sarcoidosis. (See Appendix I.) Sarcoidosis is a serious but rare inflammatory disorder that may at first manifest few if any signs. But as it progresses, sarcoidosis can affect many body parts, including the skin, eyes, ears, nose, and internal organs.

Facial, body, or limb numbness is also one of the most common and earliest warning signs of the neuromuscular disorder *multiple sclerosis (MS).* In addition, paresthesia

SIGNIFICANT FACT

A recent British study found that women with ring fingers that are longer than their index fingers—usually a male trait—were better at such sports as running, tennis, and soccer than other women. But, according to an Australian study, they're also at increased risk for *polycystic ovary syndrome (PCOS),* a common cause of infertility. The scientists attribute both the athletic ability and PCOS to overexposure to male hormones in the womb.

SIGN OF THE TIMES

Doctors are seeing more and more *repetitive-stress injuries (RSIs)* from using personal digital assistants (PDAs). Dubbed "BlackBerry thumb," this condition causes pain and/or numbness in the thumb or finger joints. Even those too young to own a BlackBerry aren't exempt. Many children are falling victim to "video-gamer's thumb," aka "Nintendo thumb"—a type of RSI caused by playing with PlayStations or other video games.

can be a clue to *vitamin B$_{12}$ deficiency* or even the more serious *pernicious anemia,* a severe form of anemia (low red blood cell count) caused by the body's inability to absorb vitamin B$_{12}$. Interestingly, too much vitamin B$_6$ can cause paresthesia, as can abnormally high levels of calcium, potassium, sodium, and lead. Excessive tobacco and alcohol use can produce numbness and/or tingliness, too.

WARNING SIGNS

Sudden numbness or tingliness along with any of the following may signal either a mini-stroke—medically called a *transient ischemic attack (TIA)*—or a full-blown stroke:

- Weakness in an arm or leg, face, or one side of your body
- Having trouble speaking, seeing, or walking
- Dizziness or fainting
- Confusion or difficulty understanding people
- Sudden headache, especially with a stiff neck

NUMB OR TINGLY EXTREMITIES

Numb or tingly legs, in particular, are sometimes signs of *peripheral arterial disease (PAD)*; also called *peripheral vascular disease,* or *PVD,* a serious circulatory problem that affects arteries other than in the heart and brain. PAD is caused by a buildup of fatty plaque in the legs, much like the fat deposits seen in the heart in *coronary artery disease (CAD)* or the brain in *cerebrovascular disease.* And like people with CAD, people with PAD are at very increased risk of heart attacks and strokes.

Some other PAD signs are leg cramps when walking and coldness in the extremities. (See **Leg Cramps During the Day** and **Cold Hands and Feet,** below.) Having diabetes increases the risk of PAD. And because diabetes itself can lead to heart disease, stroke, and decreased circulation in the legs and feet, having both PAD and diabetes raises the risk of these complications as well as foot and leg amputations.

Numbness and tingling in the arms or legs can also be early warning signs of *peripheral neuropathy (PN)*—damage to the *peripheral nervous system,* the nerves that transmit sensory signals to and from the brain and spinal cord. As PN progresses, feeling in the arms, fingers, legs, and toes diminishes, increasing the risk of infections, wounds that don't heal, and consequent amputations. Uncontrolled diabetes is a leading cause of peripheral neuropathy in the United States.

A physical injury, an autoimmune disorder, or a bacterial or viral infection—such as shingles, *Lyme disease* (a bacterial infection transmitted by deer ticks), or HIV/AIDS—can also cause nerve damage. PN-related numbness and tingling can signal a whole host of systemic disorders ranging from vitamin deficiencies to kidney disease, hormonal imbalances, diabetes, alcohol addiction, and benign or cancerous tumors. It can also be a reaction to some of the drugs used to treat cancer.

SIGNIFICANT FACT

About 75% of people with peripheral artery disease don't have any signs, so the condition goes undiagnosed. And women are less likely than men to have PAD signs.

Numb or tingly arms or legs can signal *hyperaldosteronism,* an excess of the hormone aldosterone, which is made by the adrenal glands and helps maintain the salt and water balance in your body. Besides leading to numbness and tingliness, too much aldosterone can cause you to retain sodium and lose potassium, resulting in frequent urination, muscle weakness or cramps, and high blood pressure. Hyperaldosteronism itself can signal an adrenal tumor known as *Conn's syndrome.* The good news is that this tumor is noncancerous in 95% of cases.

SIGN OF THE TIMES

In the 1986 book *No Laughing Matter,* Joseph Heller, best known for his best-selling novel *Catch-22,* chronicled his paralysis and recovery from *Guillain-Barré syndrome.*

Lastly, tingliness—particularly in the legs—is one of the earliest signs of *Guillain-Barré syndrome,* a potentially life-threatening disorder. This progressive and sometimes rapid-onset disease causes the body's immune system to attack the peripheral nervous system, leading to paralysis. Guillain-Barré syndrome can occur after a viral infection, surgery, or trauma, or as a reaction to an immunization.

THAT FUNNY-BONE FEELING

If you've ever banged your elbow, you know what hitting your funny bone feels like. You also know it's far from funny; it may feel like an electric, tingly shock up and down your arm. But if you have this feeling even when you haven't whacked your elbow, you probably have what's medically known as *cubital tunnel syndrome*, a nerve compression disorder. In both cases it's the ulnar nerve that's being affected, and the funny sensations can spread from the elbow to the hand and the fingers—usually the pinky and ring finger. The funny-bone sensation is usually a clue that you've had your elbow flexed for long periods, such as during sleep. Or it may mean that you were working at a computer, engaging in activities that involve repeatedly bending the elbow (such as doing biceps curls), or have had an injury to your elbow. While cubital tunnel syndrome is usually benign, in severe cases the muscles in the forearm may weaken.

> ### SIGN OF THE TIMES
>
> Some attribute the term *funny bone*—which used to be called *crazy bone*—to the 19th-century poet Reverend Richard Harris Barham, known for his puns. The bone involved is the large knob (*medial condyle*) at the end of the bone of the upper arm (*humerus*).

Cubital tunnel syndrome is similar to golfer's elbow—medically known as *medial epicondylitis*—but people with golfer's elbow usually complain more of pain than tingling.

TINGLY, NUMB FINGERS

Sometimes that all-too-familiar funny-bone feeling is felt in the fingers or even the feet rather than the elbow. Tingly, numb, and sometimes burning fingers may point to *carpal tunnel syndrome,* a nerve condition caused by pressure on the *median nerve* in the wrist. At first, you might think that your hand keeps falling asleep. Carpal tunnel syndrome tends to strike people in their mid-40s, and women are more apt to develop it than men. This condition is more annoying than painful, but as it progresses, the sufferer may have difficulty gripping and may frequently drop objects.

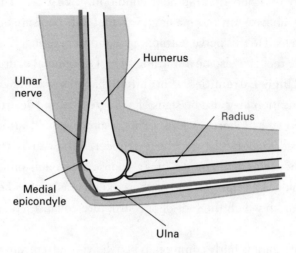

ARM AND ELBOW ANATOMY

WARNING SIGN

If you spend many hours at the computer, you probably perform between 50,000 and 200,000 keystrokes a day. This can make you vulnerable to muscle, nerve, and other injuries to your neck, back, shoulders,
arms, and hands.

It's long been believed that carpal tunnel syndrome is a sign of overuse of the fingers from activities such as typing, assembly-line work, or
piano playing. Some researchers believe, however, these factors are over-
stated; recent studies have found that in certain cases carpal tunnel syndrome can be a signal of such medical disorders as osteoarthritis (see
Creaky Knees, above), diabetes, and hypothyroidism (see **Feeling Cold
All Over,** below, and Appendix I).

TINGLY, NUMB FEET

If your feet often feel numb and tingly, it can be an indication that you're
heading toward *tarsal tunnel syndrome,* the lower-extremity cousin of
carpal tunnel syndrome (see **Tingly, Numb Fingers,** above). A hot, burning sensation in the feet is another sign of this problem, which falls under

the category of a nerve entrapment condition. (See **Body Tingling and Numbness,** above.) Any trauma or growth that puts pressure on a nerve in the foot can lead to this nerve entrapment condition. A tingly, burning sensation in the feet can also be a warning sign of peripheral neuropathy (see **Numb or Tingly Extremities,** above) from diabetes or other conditions.

This sensation may also be signs of a progressive and destructive bone disorder known as *Charcot's joint.* This disorder usually affects weight-bearing joints, in particular the knees and feet, but it can involve the hips as well. Other signs of Charcot's joint are loose or swollen joints and other foot and ankle deformities. One of these, known as *rocker bottom foot,* is a condition in which the foot's bone structure collapses, leaving a ball-like bulge.

Charcot's joint is fairly common in people who suffer from nerve damage from uncontrolled diabetes (*diabetic neuropathy*). (See **Numb or Tingly Extremities,** above.) Actually, anyone who suffers from any type of nerve damage from any cause can find themselves with this disorder.

Tingling, burning, and numbness located in the front of the foot can also be a sign of a benign lesion known as a *neuroma.* People who have this condition notice the symptoms even more when they wear a tight-fitting shoe, as the neuroma or nerve ball is compressed. Some patients will also describe the sensation of having a pebble in their shoe or the sensation that their sock is bunched up in the front. Fortunately, most neuromas can be treated successfully without surgery but may require a prescription foot orthotic or injections.

NIGHT JERKS

Ahhh . . . the sweetness of deep sleep after an exhausting day—that is, until you're jerked awake by a sudden feeling of falling. Tagged with several medical monikers—including *myoclonus, myoclonic twitch,* and *hypnic* or *hypnogogic jerk*—this is a common and benign, albeit sometimes very heart-stopping, sign. Whatever it's called, it's actually an involuntary muscle twitch that generally occurs during the transition between wakefulness and sleep. Most of us have them occasionally, and they tend to occur when we're overly tired or sleep-deprived.

These nocturnal jerks may be associated with *restless leg syndrome (RLS)*, a neurological condition (see **Jittery Legs,** below), and other sleep-related disorders.

Sometimes, however, you might be awakened repeatedly by night jerks. These movements are a bona fide medical condition called *periodic limb movement disorder (PLMD)*. PLMD can sometimes be a sign of the sleep disorder *narcolepsy,* a condition in which people fall asleep involuntarily.

JITTERY LEGS

Okay, you finally get to sit down in front of the television for a little R&R before going to bed. Suddenly you experience a searing, tingling, bubbling, "creepy-crawly" sensation in your leg, which seems to be relieved only by moving it. You're experiencing the classic signs of a neurological disorder called *restless leg syndrome (RSL)*. Although these jerky sensations, which occur at intervals of 30 to 60 seconds, can occur during both sleep and wakefulness, they strike primarily in the evening or during periods of inactivity. In fact, restless leg syndrome is sometimes considered a sleep disorder. Because the sensations can cause difficulty falling or staying asleep, RSL sufferers often feel daytime fatigue.

STOP SIGN

The Sleep Research Society and the American Academy of Sleep Medicine have devised a single question to determine which patients are likely to have restless leg syndrome: "When you try to relax in the evening or sleep at night, do you ever have unpleasant, restless feelings in your legs that can be relieved by walking or movement?" If you answer yes, you probably have this annoying condition.

RLS isn't just an impediment to getting a good night's sleep; a recent Canadian study found some evidence that it's associated with an increased risk of developing cardiovascular disease, especially in the elderly. Another study suggests that RLS and irritable bowel syndrome (see Chapter 8) may be linked.

LEG CRAMPS DURING THE NIGHT

You're peacefully in slumberland and suddenly you're awakened by a piercing sensation in your leg. You have the classic sign of *nocturnal leg cramps,* aka a *charley horse.* These involuntary contractions of calf muscles, and occasionally muscles on the soles of the feet, are very common in older people. In fact, about 70% of adults older than 50 are occasionally jolted out of sleep by these tightening sensations. People with flat feet seem to get them more often, too. While no one is quite sure what brings these night visitors on, they can be a sign of overexertion or dehydration. Although harmless, nocturnal leg cramps can sometimes signal diabetes, Parkinson's disease, anemia, and thyroid problems.

LEG CRAMPS DURING THE DAY

If you frequently get leg cramps when walking or climbing, you may be experiencing *intermittent claudication,* a decreased flow of oxygen-rich blood to the extremities caused by fatty plaque buildup in the leg arteries. This condition is the classic sign of *peripheral arterial disease (PAD),* a progressive circulatory problem that's potentially life-threatening. (See **Numb or Tingly Extremities,** above.)

DANGER SIGN

 If you have tenderness, swelling, redness, or warmth in one leg and then begin to have chest pain or trouble breathing, these can be signs of a pulmonary embolism—a potentially fatal complication of a deep vein thrombosis.

SIGN OF THE TIMES

 The term *claudication* has its roots in the Latin verb *claudi-care,* "to limp." The Roman emperor Claudius was given this name because he hobbled.

Leg cramps, particularly in one leg, can also be a sign of another potentially life-threatening condition, *deep vein thrombosis (DVT).* In DVT a clot forms in a large vein and can easily break off and travel to the heart and lungs, leading to death. Other signs of DVT, which usually come on fairly suddenly, are muscle tenderness or deep muscle pain, swelling, tenderness, warmth, and discoloration of the affected area.

DVTs occur more often in people over age 40 and those who are immobilized for a prolonged length of time from either illness, injury, or some other reason. In fact, DVT is sometimes called *economy-class syndrome* or *traveler's thrombosis* because long flights in confined coach cabins have led to DVT-related fatalities. Being cooped up causes blood to pool in the legs' deep veins, setting the stage for dangerous clotting.

SIGN OF THE TIMES

While covering the war in Iraq in 2003, NBC News correspondent David Bloom, 39, died from a pulmonary embolism caused by a clot that formed in his leg (DVT), then broke off and entered his lungs. Bloom had complained of leg cramps while riding for long hours in the narrow confines of a converted army tank.

STOP SIGN

No matter how long or short your plane flight is, get up and walk around periodically. This can help ward off DVT. Wearing support stockings or socks, especially on long flights, can also help prevent this potentially deadly condition.

Women on hormone replacement therapy or those taking birth control pills are at increased risk of developing these deadly clots, as are pregnant women. People with clotting disorders or certain medical conditions that restrict mobility, such as heart failure or chronic respiratory disease, are at risk as well.

WARNING SIGN

DVT without an obvious precipitating cause may be one of the very earliest clues to cancer. In fact, the link between DVT and cancer was first noted by the 19th-century physician Armand Trousseau. Ironically, Trousseau himself later developed DVT and was diagnosed with stomach cancer within a year.

Also at high risk for developing these clots are people with broken legs, those undergoing surgery (especially orthopedic, pelvic, or abdominal operations), and cancer patients. And if you've had one episode of DVT, you're at increased risk of having another.

TREMORS

If you notice someone's hands or body is trembling, you might assume that the person is nervous or has a drinking problem, and you may be right. But tremors can also signal a myriad of other maladies.

There are more than 20 different types of tremors. *Essential tremors* (aka *postural tremors*) are the mildest and the most common type. They usually affect the hands, but the head, arms, legs, larynx (voice box), and even the tongue can be affected as well. (See Chapter 5.)

Previously called *senile tremors* because they are common in older people, essential tremors can begin at any age. They do tend, however, to worsen as one gets older. In about half the cases, essential tremors run in families and are referred to as *familial tremors.* In the other half, the cause is unknown (idiopathic).

Although medically benign, essential tremors are frequently embarrassing and can make activities requiring fine finger movements—such as sewing, fly tying, and surgery—difficult, if not impossible. Thus, they interfere not only with quality of life but with careers as well. Interestingly, essential tremors tend to stop when the affected body part is at rest.

WARNING SIGN

 A "pill-rolling" finger gesture is a unique sign of Parkinson's disease. The tremor looks like the thumb and forefinger are rolling a pill between them. This repetitive gesture can occur as often as 3 times per second. It is most noticeable when the hand is at rest or the person is under stress.

Some tremors are drug-induced and can be a tip-off to the overuse or abuse of caffeine, nicotine, tranquilizers, amphetamines, and cocaine. And morning tremors are a dead giveaway for alcohol abuse. Tremors are also a common reaction to antipsychotic drugs, theophylline (for asthma), Dilantin (for epilepsy), and Compazine (a tranquilizer and antinausea medicine), as well as the herbal stimulants ephedra, ginkgo biloba, and ginseng.

Tremors sometimes signal *alkalosis,* a pH imbalance (too little acid in body fluids). Other signs may include muscle twitching, light-headedness, numbness, and tingling. Alkalosis-related tremors can be a clue to the eating disorder bulimia. The good news is that alkalosis is easily treated. The bad news is that if untreated, it can lead to *arrhythmias (irregular heartbeat),* coma, and possibly death.

SIGN OF THE TIMES

Several famous political figures, including Samuel Adams, Oliver Cromwell, and more recently Sandra Day O'Connor, have suffered from essential tremors. Playwright Eugene O'Neill and actress Katharine Hepburn both suffered from them as well. Indeed, Hepburn's tremulous voice was her trademark.

Tremors can also signal systemic disorders such as hypoglycemia (in both diabetics and others) and hyperthyroidism. (See **Feeling Hot When It's Not,** below, and Appendix I.) And they can signal multiple sclerosis, kidney and liver disease, stroke, or even a brain tumor.

Another type of tremor occurs when your arm, leg, or other body part is at rest. Aptly named a *resting tremor,* this is one of the earliest signs of Parkinson's disease. Other early signs of Parkinson's may include a change in handwriting, loss of sense of smell (see Chapter 4), stumbling, and rigid posture.

SIGNIFICANT FACT

Our bodies are vibrating continuously. The only time we're perfectly still is when we're dead.

FEELING YOUR HEART BEAT

Most of us are unaware of the beating of our hearts unless we've been running or exercising. But some of us notice a strong, fast, fluttering, or irregular heartbeat even when we're still. This may be more noticeable when lying down, particularly on our left side. This awareness of our heart beating—medically known as *palpitations*—is usually a normal, benign sensation. The term *palpitation* is commonly used to describe irregular, in particular, fast, heartbeats, too.

Palpitations are a common sign of everyday anxiety and fear—the typical flight-or-fight reaction. But they can be severe, too, as in a *panic attack.* A racing, pounding heart can also be a clue that you've been smoking, drinking too much alcohol, or consuming too much caffeine from coffee, tea, or colas. Palpitations can also signal cocaine or amphetamine abuse, or they can be a reaction to some common drugs that cause tremors (see **Tremors,** above), such as some decongestants, antidepressants, asthma medicines, and thyroid medications. Certain herbal supplements, such as ginseng, and those touted for weight loss, such as guarana and ephedra, can also make your heart race.

Palpitations can signal a plethora of medical problems as well. They can, for example, be a sign of a fever, anemia, low blood sugar (*hypoglycemia*), low potassium levels, or hyperthyroidism. (See **Feeling Hot When It's Not**, below, and Appendix I.)

Not surprisingly, palpitations are a common sign of both benign and serious heart problems. These include *mitral valve prolapse* (a very common and usually not too serious heart valve deformity) and *arrhythmias,* abnormal or irregular heartbeats. Indeed, the terms *palpitation* and *arrhythmia* are often used interchangeably. When the heart beats too fast, it's referred to as *tachycardia;* when it beats too slow, it's called *bradycardia.*

SPEAKING OF SIGNS

The heart is not a Swiss watch, but a complex biologic system that suffers from occasional hiccups.

—Douglas Zipes, MD, cardiologist, Indiana University School of Medicine

If you feel an extra beat, it can be a sign of *premature atrial contractions (PACs),* the most common and benign type of arrhythmia. On the other hand, if you feel like your heart occasionally skips a beat, it may be a sign of *premature ventricular contractions (PVCs).* While PVCs are often benign, they can be a sign of heart disease or an electrolyte imbalance—an imbalance of minerals in the blood that can cause serious heart and kidney problems if untreated. Unfortunately, some PVCs are potentially life-threatening, especially when accompanied by a racing heart, dizziness, or fainting, or in a person with heart disease.

TEMPERAMENTAL TEMPERATURES

COLD HANDS AND FEET

When people shake your hand, do they often comment on your cold hands? And does the thought of going barefoot cause a shudder? We all suffer from cold hands and feet at some point, usually in winter or in overly air-conditioned rooms. But if your extremities are chronically cold, it can be a reaction to certain drugs such as beta-blockers, thyroid medications, and drugs used to treat migraines.

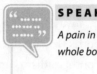

SPEAKING OF SIGNS

A pain in the little finger is felt by the whole body.

—Philippine proverb

Cold fingers and toes that turn blue or white when exposed to the cold are the hallmark of *Raynaud's disease* (aka *Raynaud's phenomenon*), a circulatory disorder in which the blood supply to the hands and feet is reduced. Exposure to cold temperatures can precipitate an attack, but in some people stress can do so as well. Typically, fingers and toes not only turn colors, they may throb or feel tingly or numb. Earlobes, noses, and legs are sometimes affected also.

SPEAKING OF SIGNS

The chief function of the body is to carry the brain around.

—Thomas A. Edison

Raynaud's affects about 5 to 10% of people in the United States and is more likely to occur in women between the ages of 20 and 40 and in smokers. Unfortunately, in women, Raynaud's sometimes goes hand in hand with *fibromyalgia,* a physically incapacitating musculoskeletal condition that also tends to strike more women than men. About 30% of people with fibromyalgia also have Raynaud's.

Cold hands and feet can also signal *peripheral arterial disease (PAD).* (See **Numb or Tingly Extremities,** above.) And it can signal the potentially serious condition *Buerger's disease,* also known as thrombo-angiitis. This rare condition is almost exclusively seen in men between the ages of 20 and 40 who smoke or chew tobacco. In both PAD and Buerger's disease, fatty deposits build up in the arteries and restrict blood circulation to the stomach, kidneys, arms, legs, hands, and feet *(athero-sclerosis).* Other signs include color changes in legs, problems walking, and *erectile dysfunction* (impotence). As with PAD, Buerger's disease can lead to gangrene and necessitate amputation.

FEELING COLD ALL OVER

Do you find that you're always putting on a sweater and turning the heat up when others are perfectly comfortable? If so, you may have one of the telltale signs of hypothyroidism, an underactive thyroid gland, which produces too little thyroid hormone. (See Appendix I.) Although hypothyroidism affects both sexes, it's especially common, but very often misdiagnosed, in adult and elderly women. Other typical signs include weight gain, dry skin, hoarse voice, and constipation.

SIGNIFICANT FACT

The elderly often feel cold even in the summer, and they tend to avoid fans and air-conditioning. As a result, they're very susceptible to heat stroke and heat-related heart attacks. Indeed, 35,000 people, most of whom were elderly, died during a record heat wave in Europe in 2003.

Cold intolerance can also signal the hormone-related disorder *hypopituitarism,* a malfunction of the pituitary, the endocrine system's master gland. In addition to hypersensitivity to cold, people with hypopituitarism may suffer from fatigue, fertility problems, and low blood pressure. And cold intolerance can be a sign of another hormone-related disorder, *hypothalamic dysfunction,* which affects the hypothalamus, a gland that helps regulate body temperature, appetite, weight, and emotions. Hypothalamic dysfunction can itself be a sign of a tumor, infection, head trauma, or malnutrition.

Feeling cold much of the time can also be a sign that you're anemic. About 20% of people with iron-deficiency anemia suffer from cold intolerance. On rare occasions, sensitivity to cold can be a warning sign of bone cancer or *leukemia* (cancer of the blood and blood marrow).

If you feel cold a lot, as well as stiff and achy, you may have *fibromyalgia* (see **Cold Hands and Feet,** above), a musculoskeletal condition that also tends to strike women. While not life-threatening, it can be incapacitating.

FEELING HOT WHEN IT'S NOT

Who hasn't heard the menopause mantra "Is it hot in here or is it me?" Feeling hot a lot and having hot flashes are telltale signs of menopause, but not all women who complain of heat intolerance are having menopause-related hot flashes. And not all heat-intolerance sufferers are women. Heat intolerance is a classic sign of several hormone-related conditions, especially *hyperthyroidism,* in which excess thyroid hormone raises your temperature and speeds up your metabolism. (See Appendix I.) Other common signs are nervousness, weight loss, excessive hunger and thirst, and bulging eyes. While both men and women can suffer from an overactive thyroid, it's more prevalent among women.

Feeling hot a lot can be a reaction to excess caffeine, amphetamines, certain antidepressants, and thyroid medication. And sensitivity to heat may even signal such serious conditions as multiple sclerosis (MS). Indeed, exposure to heat and hot water can temporarily worsen MS symptoms, which include tremors, blurred vision, and memory problems. Heat intolerance can also be a red flag for *anhidrosis,* the inability to sweat. This can be a life-threatening condition. (See Chapter 8.) People who don't sweat can get so overheated, they're at increased risk of heat exhaustion and heat stroke.

SIGNING OFF

There are a myriad of body parts in and on the torso, and there are an almost infinite number of things that can go awry with any of them. Below is a list of specialists who might help. However, if you're experiencing chronic or extreme pain, bleeding, vomiting, excessive or sudden swelling, intense itching, dizziness, or fainting, start with an immediate visit to your primary care physician or to the emergency room.

- *Cardiologist:* A medical doctor who specializes in diagnosing and treating diseases and disorders of the heart and circulatory system.
- *Endocrinologist:* A medical doctor who specializes in diagnosing and treating hormone-related diseases and disorders.
- *Gynecologist:* A medical doctor who specializes in diagnosing and treating conditions related to the female reproductive system. Some gynecologists also perform surgery.
- *Neurologist:* A medical doctor who specializes in diseases and disorders related to the central nervous system (the brain and spinal cord) and the peripheral nervous system (the sensory and motor nerves).
- *Oncologist:* A medical doctor who specializes in treating cancer. Some oncologists also perform surgery or further specialize in treating cancer with radiation therapy.
- *Orthopedist:* A medical doctor and surgeon who specializes in the treatment of diseases and disorders of the bones, joints, and muscles.
- *Podiatrist:* A doctor of podiatric medicine (DPM) who specializes in the treatment of diseases and disorders of the foot and ankle. (In England, they're known as chiropodists.)
- *Physical Therapist:* A health care professional specially trained to evaluate and treat problems of physical mobility and muscle function.
- *Rheumatologist:* A medical doctor who specializes in diagnosing and treating diseases and disorders involving the joints, muscles, tendons, ligaments, connective tissue, and bones.

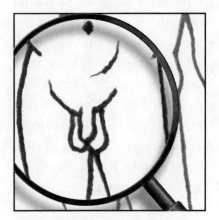

CHAPTER 8

PRIVATE PARTS, FARTS, AND BODY WASTES

Let not thy privy members be
layd open to be view'd
it is most shameful and
   abhord
detestable and rude.

—RICHARD WESTE, 1619

Private parts weren't always considered shameful—or even all
that private, for that matter.
Indeed, when Adam and Eve first inhab-
ited the Garden of Eden, "they were
both naked...and they were not
ashamed," according to the Bible. But a
bit later, after they bit that notorious apple, they became aware of their
nakedness, and the fig leaf became humankind's first fashion fad.

Since then, nudity and shame have gone hand in hand. Despite the
stigma sometimes attached to our genitals, the fascination with our own
and others' has endured. Throughout history, depictions of frontal and
rear nudity have graced the walls of caves, museums, bedrooms, bath-
rooms, barrooms, and bordellos.

Part of our obsession with—and ambivalence about—our private
parts is not only the pleasure they can give us and others but also the fact
that they're necessary for both procreation and elimination. Because we

make love and babies with our genitals and urine comes out of them as well, they both attract and repel. And we haven't even touched on the buttocks and their end product.

Some of our body wastes (or *humors,* as some were called) have been the subject of study, and humor, for thousands of years. Hippocrates, often known as the Father of Medicine, taught that there were four humors, which affected both physical and mental health: yellow bile, black bile, blood, and phlegm. All diseases were thought to stem from an imbalance of these "essential fluids" and the body's consequent inability to rid itself of its waste products. The cures: sweating, purging, bloodletting, and vomiting.

SPEAKING OF SIGNS

To hear many religious people talk, one would think God created the torso, head, legs and arms, but the devil slapped on the genitals.

—Don Schrader, TV personality and cultural commentator in New Mexico

SPEAKING OF SIGNS

The sex organ of a man is simple and neat as a finger, but the female sex organ is mysterious even to the woman herself, concealed, mucous, and humid.

—Simone de Beauvoir, *The Second Sex,* 1949

Today, we still spend an inordinate amount of time and money trying to eliminate our body wastes. While bloodletting and induced vomiting are not for everyone, many of us occasionally purge with laxatives or enemas, take diuretics, or sweat it out in saunas and gyms. And leeches are back in vogue, too.

Our reproductive, digestive, urinary, and body-temperature regulating systems are wonders of nature but can also produce a myriad of disconcerting—and downright embarrassing—smells, sounds, and sights. Penises, for example, come in a wide variety of sizes, shapes, and colors that seem to change magically throughout the day and night. While vaginas are sometimes seen, they're seldom heard—that is, unless a woman suffers from vaginal farts. And the stomach and intestines can produce an astounding array of not very melodious sounds, often accompanied by malodorous smells.

And let's not forget sweat, the most neglected of our body wastes—at least when it comes to bathroom humor and slang terms. But sweat takes first prize for sticking around. Unlike poop and pee, which can easily be flushed away and forgotten, the smell of sweat can long linger on our bodies and clothes and in gyms and taxis without the help of soap and water to wash it away.

The body signs related to our private parts and their often disagreeable by-products are major sources of humor to many kids and adults alike. But because they're also a major source of embarrassment, we may find these body waste signs difficult to discuss with

SIGNIFICANT FACT

Some scientists believe that the strong body odors that accompany some diseases may have evolved as a way of warning people away from potentially diseased mates.

our doctors. That can be a big mistake. Whether you're a fan of bathroom humor or not, you shouldn't ignore the body signs that your internal waste management system periodically spews out at you. Embarrassing or not, they can reveal countless clues about the state of our bodies. Studying your stools, urine, sweat, and other body wastes is definitely *not* a waste of time. The lessons learned can be invaluable or even life-saving.

SIGN OF THE TIMES

The 16th-century German theologian Martin Luther claimed he could "drive away the evil spirit with a single fart."

PENILE PECULIARITIES

CROOKED PENIS

While some men may have a bent for certain sexual practices, some actually have a bent sex organ. Although a crooked penis can be a perfectly benign anatomical anomaly (medically known as *congenital penile curvature*), it's sometimes a sign of *Peyronie's disease (PD)*. (See Chapter 7.) In this condition, a hard lump or patches (*plaque*) beneath the skin form on the penile shaft, forcing it to turn up, down, left, or right. PD can pop up overnight or gradually and can sometimes be extremely painful, making sexual intercourse difficult or even impossible. Many men are very embarrassed by this condition, compounding their sexual problems.

Also known as *fibrous cavernositis,* Peyronie's disease occasionally runs in families. But it's more likely a sign of physical trauma to the penis, possibly from a sports injury or even overly vigorous sex. It can also signal *vasculitis,* an inflammation of blood or lymphatic vessels. About 30% of men with PD also have *connective tissue disorders*. The most common is *Dupuytren's disease,* an abnormal thickening of the skin on the palms of the hands that causes the fingers— much like the penis in PD—to curl. (See Chapter 7.)

SIGN OF THE TIMES

The 18th-century French surgeon François Gigot de Peyronie reported three cases of the penile disorder that now bears his name. However, the first professional to write about Peyronie's disease was the 16th-century Italian anatomist and surgeon, Giulio Cesare Aranzi. He described this disorder as "a rare affliction of the genitals in people with excessive sexual intercourse." Former U.S. president Bill Clinton is said to have this condition.

Peyronie's disease tends to affect men between the ages of 40 and 60 and is more prevalent among whites than blacks or Asians. Up to 4% of white men in the United States are affected. The typical patient is an older man who has weak erections but who engages in energetic, frequent (more than four times a week) intercourse. The good news is that PD can disappear on its own. But occasionally surgery is needed to correct this condition, especially if it continues to cause pain or sexual problems.

A PROLONGED ERECTION

It may sound like every man's—and some women's—dream. But an erection that lasts longer than four hours without continued sexual stimulation is a sign of *priapism,* which can be uncomfortable, embarrassing, and even painful. It can also lead to permanent organ damage.

Priapism is very common in men with sickle-cell anemia; indeed, about 42% of men who have this condition will suffer from priapism at some point in their lives. (It's also a common reaction to an uncommon event, a black widow spider bite. But you'd be more likely to be aware of the severe pain and muscle cramping the bite can cause.) Less commonly, prolonged erections can signal **leukemia** or **malaria**.

Prolonged erections can also be a reaction to certain antipsychotics, as well as some antidepressants and antihypertensives. And not surprisingly, they can be a rare overreaction to such drugs as Viagra, Cialis, and Levitra, which are used to treat **erectile dysfunction (ED)**, commonly called impotence. Priapism can also be a sign of carbon monoxide poisoning as well as alcohol, marijuana, cocaine, and other drug abuse. In addition, it can signal a spinal cord injury or disease, as well as an injury to the penis. Priapism is considered a medical emergency that, if untreated, can lead to serious scarring and permanent ED.

SIGN OF THE TIMES

Priapism was named after Priapus, the Greek god of gardening and fertility, and son of Aphrodite. So homely a baby was he that the gods tossed him off Mt. Olympus and he was raised among the nymphs and satyrs. One day his penis grew so large and heavy he couldn't move. To add insult to injury, he had a permanent erection but couldn't ejaculate.

WARNING SIGN

Erectile dysfunction (ED) may be the earliest warning sign of heart disease. In fact, according to some recent studies, coronary heart disease tends to crop up about 3 years after the ED. The more severe the ED, the more serious the heart disease.

SPOTTED PENIS

If your partner dons a colored condom, you might find it funny, if not sexy. But if his penis itself has changed color, it's not a laughing matter. A reddish or purplish painless ulcer on the penis is usually the earliest warning sign of **penile cancer**, a rare form of skin cancer mostly found in uncircumcised men. As the cancer progresses, other signs, such as a red rash and a foul-smelling discharge, or bleeding, sometimes occur.

Men infected with the **human papillomavirus (HPV)**—one of the most common **sexually transmitted diseases (STDs)** in men and women—are at considerably higher risk of cancer of the penis than other men. Men who smoke, have HIV/AIDS, or have been treated for psoriasis with ultraviolet light and the drug psoralen are at increased risk of penile cancer, too.

SCROTAL SWELLING

If a man notices a soft swelling within his scrotum, it may give him pause, or he may not even give it a second thought. In fact, it's probably nothing to worry about. This type of intrascrotal swelling is most likely a sign of a *varicocele,* which is actually a varicose vein surrounding the testicle and similar to a varicose vein on the leg. (See Chapter 9.) Usually found around the left testicle (although they can occur around both), varicoceles are noticed more easily when a man is standing and they tend to disappear when he reclines. Some men say that varicoceles feel like having "a bag of worms" within their scrotal sac.

SPEAKING OF SIGNS

The three most important things a man has are, briefly, his private parts, his money, and his religious opinions.

—Samuel Butler, 19th-century English writer

SIGNIFICANT FACT

About half of newborn baby boys have hydroceles. These scrotal swellings usually disappear by the baby's first birthday.

Approximately 15 to 20% of men have varicoceles, and they're most common in men between the ages of 15 and 25. Although usually benign, they can be warning signs of infertility: as many as 40% of men with fertility problems have varicoceles. It's believed that a varicocele can interfere with sperm production by increasing the temperature of the testicles.

Scrotal swelling can also be a sign of a *hydrocele,* a painless buildup of fluid around a testicle that usually develops after age 40. It can signal a scrotal injury or infection. A hydrocele can be confused with an *inguinal hernia,* a condition in which part of the intestine protrudes through a weakened abdominal wall into the scrotum. (See Chapter 9.) Occasionally, a hydrocele can signal testicular cancer. (See **A Lump on the Testicle,** below.)

Scrotal swelling—as well as heavy-feeling testicles—can also be a sign of a serious infection of the *epididymis,* the spiral tube that stores and helps transport sperm. Medically called *epididymitis,* this infection is usually caused by an STD, such as chlamydia or gonorrhea. Although scrotal swelling and penile discharge are fairly common with epididymitis, the first thing men will likely notice is the discomfort, which can range from mild to very severe. (See **Penile Discharge,** below.) Epididymitis can also be a reaction to amiodarone, a drug used to treat heart rhythm disturbances. Lastly, epididymitis can signal tuberculosis.

SPEAKING OF SIGNS

If the head is lost, all that perishes is the individual; if the balls are lost, all human nature perishes.

—François Rabelais,
16th-century French author

If the whole scrotum is swollen but not painful, it can be a sign of *lymphedema,* which is a condition that primarily affects the arms and legs. (See Chapter 9.) It can be caused by a blockage in the lymphatic system that prevents lymph fluids (which collect viruses, bacteria, and waste products from the body) from draining. Lymphedema itself is often a serious warning sign of heart failure or cirrhosis of the liver.

A SWOLLEN PENIS HEAD

Probably we've all met a few men with swollen heads. But if the head of a man's penis (*glans penis*) is swollen, he may have nothing to be proud about. Rather, he may be sporting a medical condition called *balanitis,* a sign that he's not practicing good personal hygiene. He may even have a smelly discharge. If a man's not circumcised, his foreskin (*prepuce*) may also become inflamed—a condition called *posthitis.* Ultimately, inflammation and swelling can become so bad that an uncircumcised man can't pull back his foreskin, a condition medically known as *phimosis.*

A LUMP ON THE TESTICLE

Finding a lump on your testicle can put a lump in your throat. But a painless lump may merely be a sign of a *spermatocele,* a benign cyst-like collection of sperm within the scrotum but attached to the epididymis. Or it can signal a testicular injury or infection.

Unfortunately, sometimes a firm, painless lump can be a marker for *testicular cancer*; in fact, it's the most common sign. Other possible signs include a heaviness or discomfort in the scrotum; a dull ache in the groin, abdomen, or back; or enlarged or tender breasts. (See Chapter 7.) However, some men with testicular cancer have no discernible signs at all.

Testicular cancer is a rare cancer that affects primarily young men between the ages of 15 and 34; it's seldom seen in those over 40. In the United States, whites have the highest incidence, followed by Hispanics, Native Americans, and Asians; blacks have the lowest. It's more prevalent among men who were born with an *undescended testicle*, and it sometimes runs in families. Also at increased risk for testicular cancer are men born with an extra X chromosome, a genetic condition called *Klinefelter's syndrome*. (See Chapter 1.) The good news is that with early detection and treatment, survival rates for testicular cancer are very good.

SIGN OF THE TIMES

In 1996, world champion cyclist Lance Armstrong was diagnosed at age 25 with testicular cancer. Not only was his treatment successful, but he went on to establish the Lance Armstrong Foundation, a not-for-profit cancer support and education organization. And he won the Tour de France for 7 years running, from 1999 through 2005.

WARNING SIGN

All men—especially those between the ages of 15 and 35—should perform monthly testicular self-exams. The best time to check for lumps is after a warm bath or shower.
Here's how:

- Place your thumb on top of your testicle. Put your index and middle fingers under the testicle.
- Roll the testicle between the thumb and fingers.
- Feel for lumps, which can be as small as a pea.
- See a physician immediately if you feel anything of concern.

RED EJACULATE

Seeing red anything, particularly when it relates to our sex organs, can throw a scare into anyone. Red ejaculate, medically known as *hematospermia,* is usually a sign of the presence of blood in the seminal fluid. The blood could have gotten there from almost any type of inflammation along the reproductive tract. Men who've had one episode of red-stained ejaculate are likely to see red again. Although this sign is usually nothing to worry about, there is a slight increase in the incidence of prostate cancer among men who have had hemato-spermia.

PENILE DISCHARGE

When it comes to stuff coming out of the penis, if it's not semen or urine, it's probably a telltale sign of an STD or other infection. Penile discharge is often a sign of *urethritis*—inflammation of the urethra, the tube through which urine leaves the body. The urethra is a near-perfect conduit for microbes to enter and leave the penis. These germs can come from such sources as a catheter, a prostate infection, or another person during sexual activity.

> **SIGNIFICANT FACT**
>
> The thick, sticky, smelly, cheese-like substance that accumulates under the foreskin is called *smegma*. It's made up of oily secretions and dead skin cells. Ironically, the word *smegma* comes from the Greek for "soap"—A hint, perhaps?

Penile discharges are hard to miss and often easy to assign a cause to—for example, a thick, cloudy, and foul-smelling discharge is the hallmark of *gonorrhea,* aka "the clap."

VAGINAL VICISSITUDES

VAGINAL FARTS

A man may find having a bent or spotted penis embarrassing, but imagine a woman having a farting vagina! This little-discussed sign—medically known as *flatus vaginalis*—is actually more common than you might think. Vaginal farts are dubbed "queefs" and "varts" in the United States and "fanny farts" in England and Australia (where *fanny* refers to a woman's *vulva* rather than her buttocks).

Vaginal farts are usually a benign sign of sexual activity: the thrusting motion of intercourse can force air in and out of the vagina, as can oral sex. But various exercises, including yoga, can also give rise to this embarrassing sound.

WARNING SIGN

If oral sex is causing vaginal farts, have your partner switch immediately to a different technique. Air blown into the vagina can cause an air embolism, a potentially life-threatening condition. If a woman is pregnant, the life of her unborn child can also be in jeopardy.

Normally, vaginal farts are odorless. If, however, they give off a strong, unpleasant smell, it can be a warning sign of a tear between the vagina and colon (*colovaginal fistula*). These tears—which can happen during childbirth or as a result of *Crohn's Disease,* (see **Red or Maroon Stools,** below) and other gastrointestinal diseases—can cause infections, as well as other serious problems.

VAGINAL DISCHARGE

If you're a woman, you're well aware of the wet, sometimes sticky stuff that stains your underwear. This vaginal mucus is perfectly normal.

The amount and consistency of vaginal mucus changes throughout a woman's menstrual cycle, as well as her life cycle. Just prior to ovulation,

a woman's vaginal mucus becomes very clear and stretchable—a characteristic medically known as *spinnbarkeit*. During pregnancy, a small
amount of thickened mucus, known as the *mucus plug*, seals the cervical
canal; when the plug plops out, it's a sure sign that labor is close at hand.
As a woman ages, and her estrogen levels drop during menopause, her
mucus production usually diminishes.

WARNING SIGN

Not only is douching unnecessary, it can be dangerous. Douching can irritate the delicate vaginal tissues. The possible results:
- The vagina is left open to infection, such as sexually transmitted
  diseases, including HIV.
- An infection can be caused by disrupting the natural balance of
  organisms in the vagina.
- Germs can be pushed up into the reproductive organs, leading to
  serious infections and infertility.

Regardless of the amount, most vaginal discharge is normal. But unusual changes in its consistency and smell sometimes signal trouble. For
example, a thick, white discharge, often described as having a "cottage-
cheese consistency," is the hallmark of a vaginal yeast infection. Vaginal
yeast infections—medically called *vulvovaginal candidiasis* or *vaginal
candida* (aka *vaginal thrush*)—are very common in women between the
ages of 20 and 40. Other signs of
these vexing infections include
itching and discomfort when urinating, called *dysuria*. These can
also be signs of other vaginal as well
as urinary tract infections. (See
Cloudy Urine, below.) While the
discharge from a yeast infection is
often odorless, a woman can sometimes detect a yeasty smell, like that
of baking bread or beer.

HEALTHY SIGN

Normal vaginal mucus or discharge is clear or milky and
doesn't have a disagreeable
smell. Produced mainly by the cervix,
vaginal mucus is a sign that the vagina is
being well cleansed and moisturized. The
vagina becomes dry without good lubrication. This can open it up to infections
and make sexual intercourse painful.

A vaginal discharge that's white or gray but thin, particularly if it looks
frothy, can be a sign of *bacterial vaginosis (BV)*, the most common type

of vaginal infection in women of childbearing age. It's much more serious—and smelly—than yeast infections. Indeed, it frequently gives off an offensive, distinctive "fishy" odor, particularly after sex. Speaking of sex, BV is considered an STD, even though its exact cause is sometimes unknown. It occurs when the normal balance of bacteria in the vagina tips. Although having a new partner or multiple sex partners increases a woman's risk of BV, even women who aren't sexually active can get this potentially dangerous infection.

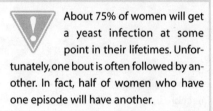

SIGNIFICANT FACT

 About 75% of women will get a yeast infection at some point in their lifetimes. Unfortunately, one bout is often followed by another. In fact, half of women who have one episode will have another.

WARNING SIGN

About 16% of pregnant women have *bacterial vaginosis,* but many don't realize it because BV doesn't always produce signs. Unfortunately, BV puts pregnant women, their babies, and their future fertility at risk. Miscarriage, premature births, low-birth-weight babies, and pelvic inflammatory disease can result from BV during pregnancy.

Yellow, frothy, smelly vaginal discharge, as well as itching and a burning sensation when urinating, can signal a microscopic parasitic infection *trichomonas vaginalis.* Commonly called "trich," this is another very common STD in the United States and in many other parts of the world.

STOMACH SOUNDS AND SMELLS

A GURGLING STOMACH

Hearing your stomach grumble, especially in a crowded room, can be mortifying. Medically known by the onomatopoeic term *borborygmus* (that's Greek for "rumbling"), these sounds, which emanate from both your stomach and intestines, are actually healthy signs that your digestive

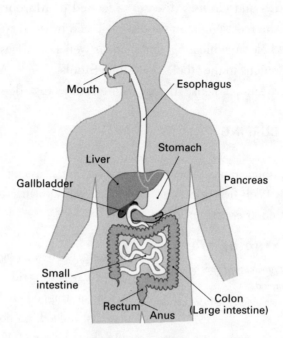

Mouth
Esophagus
Stomach
Liver
Gallbladder
Pancreas
Small intestine
Rectum
Anus
Colon (Large intestine)

DIGESTIVE SYSTEM

system is working well. They're caused by *peristalsis,* wave-like contractions of the walls of the gastrointestinal (GI) tract that help push food, fluid, and gas through the digestive system. Your stomach and intestines are constantly making noises, whether they're empty or not, but when you're full the gurgling or growling sounds are muffled.

Although usually benign, a gurgling stomach can sometimes signal serious GI problems, especially if accompanied by bloating, gas, cramps, or diarrhea. The possible problems include stomach viruses, bowel obstructions, *gastritis (inflammation of the stomach), irritable bowel syndrome (IBS, aka spastic colon),* and *inflammatory bowel disease (IBD),* which is the umbrella

> **SIGNIFICANT FACT**
>
> It's long been known that yawning as well as coughing can be contagious. Recently, London researchers found that certain other body sounds are contagious as well. They proved that the saying "Laugh and the whole world laughs with you" was quite true. However, their not-so-funny finding was that the sound of retching is contagious as well.

term for *colitis* and *Crohn's disease.* (See **Red or Maroon Stools,** below.) IBS is the most common GI disorder seen by doctors. Other signs may include belching, bloating, and pain, as well as changes in stool frequency and mucus in the stool. (See **Slimy Stools,** below.) Although IBS and IBD have similar signs, IBD is a more serious disorder.

EXCESSIVE BURPING

Burping in public comes in a close second for embarrassing body sounds. While farting takes first prize, burping—medically known as *eructation*—is really just another form of flatulence.

SPEAKING OF SIGNS

The First Amendment does not cover burping.

—Bart Simpson, TV cartoon character

For most of us, burping, aka belching, is a benign sign of stomach gas—we're getting rid of excess swallowed air trapped in our digestive systems. Indeed, it's normal to burp 3 or 4 times after a meal. Of course, burping can also be a self-induced sign of wanting to attract attention or gross out others. (Think teenage boys and fraternity brothers.)

But if you burp a lot against your will, it may be a sign of imbibing too many carbonated beverages, chewing too much gum, or eating too fast. Both burping and farting may be signs of having eaten foods high in fiber (such as beans, some fruits and vegetables, and whole grains), dairy products, artificial sweeteners, and/or carbohydrates, especially sugar and starch.

Excessive burping (and farting) can also signal a *lactase deficiency*

SIGNIFICANT FACT

According to Nebraska law, if a child burps in church, the parents can be arrested.

(aka *lactose intolerance*). Lactase is an enzyme necessary to break down *lactose* in the digestive tract. If this enzyme is missing, many foods, including milk and other dairy products, of which lactose is a major component can't be digested properly and the end result is gas.

Burping a lot is also a telltale sign of a food allergy or an upset stomach. Or it may be a sign of *gastroesophageal reflux disease (GERD)*, a potentially serious condition in which food or stomach acid backs up into the esophagus. (See Chapter 6.) It can also signal IBS. (See **A Gurgling Stomach,** above.)

Excessive burping can be evidence of some other serious intestinal or stomach disorders as well, including gastric ulcers, gallbladder disease, gallstones, and *hiatal hernia*. In all these conditions, however, other, more unsettling signs—such as nausea or vomiting, pain, and bowel changes—are likely to be present.

In addition, excessive burping can signal gallbladder disorders or even esophageal or colon cancer. Other signs of these conditions might include bloating, weight loss, vomiting blood, and bloody stools. (See **The Scoop on Poop,** below.) Finally, excessive burping with severe nausea or vomiting may be danger signs of a heart attack.

> **SIGNIFICANT FACT**
>
> Burping and farting are no laughing matters when it comes to global warming. The gas expelled by cows and other livestock is responsible for nearly 20% of methane emissions worldwide. Nitrogen-rich manure also adds to the problem. The situation is even worse in New Zealand, where a whopping 60% of greenhouse gas emissions come from livestock.

FREQUENT FARTING

Farting probably provokes more laughter and embarrassment than any other normal bodily function. Because of the sounds and smells that often accompany farts, they're hard to hide.

Excessive gas in the digestive system is medically known as *flatulence* or *flatus*. Gas can float around your intestines, causing bloating and sometimes pain. When the gas escapes through the mouth, as most of it does, it's a burp. (See **Excessive Burping,** above.) But when the gas is expelled through the anus, it's a fart.

> **SIGNIFICANT FACT**
>
> The word *fart* has been popular since Chaucer's day. It's become so widely accepted that the section on flatulence in the encyclopedic *Oxford Companion to the Body* is simply titled "Farting."

Interestingly, while the expressions "expelling gas" and "breaking wind" are sometimes used, no single medical term exists for the actual act of farting.

Most people fart an average of once an hour and produce between one and three pints of gas a day. The gas, which is usually odorless, consists primarily of carbon dioxide, oxygen, nitrogen, hydrogen, and sometimes methane. The latter two gases are flammable, which is why people can light their farts.

Luckily for us and others, smelly farts are more the exception than the rule. When they do smell bad, however, it's usually sulfur in the gas (from high-sulfur foods) that's to blame. Major culprits are such cruciferous vegetables as broccoli, cauliflower, and cabbage, as well as onions, garlic, eggs, and dairy products. Because many of these foods are also high in fiber, they can be especially bothersome—albeit very healthy.

SIGN OF THE TIMES

According to the 16th-century English writer John Audrey, the Earl of Oxford farted loudly while bowing deeply to Queen Elizabeth I. The earl was so embarrassed that he went into a self-imposed seven-year exile. Upon his return, the queen welcomed him by saying, *"My lord, I had forgot the fart."*

Also to blame are foods that contain sulfites, a form of sulfur added as a preservative. Dried prunes and other fruits are prime examples, as are baked goods, beer, wine, apple cider, and many other foods and beverages as well.

Smelly farts—and stools, for that matter—can also signal an overabundance of bacteria in the large intestine. (See **The Scoop on Poop,** below.) And speaking of stools, when the rectum is filled with them, the smell of the feces seeps out with the fart.

Frequent farting can also be a sign that you're lactose-intolerant (see **Excessive Burping,** above) or have food allergies. Or it can be an indication of some serious GI conditions such as gallstones, IBS, or IBD. (See **A Gurgling Stomach,** above.) Excess flatulence may sometimes signal cancer of the esophagus, colon, or rectum.

SIGNIFICANT FACT

For hundreds of years, cases of people bursting into flames for no apparent reason—a phenomenon known as *spontaneous combustion*—have been reported. Some scientists believe these unfortunate events are the result of static electricity igniting farts.

FEELING BLOATED

Have you ever felt like—or even looked like—you've swallowed a balloon? If so, you might actually have had a balloon of air in your stomach. Like belching and flatulence (see **Excessive Burping** and **Frequent Farting,** above), feeling bloated or having a distended stomach are often signs of excess gas. But in the case of bloating, the gas doesn't get released; the result—a swollen belly. In fact, bloating can be a sign of the same conditions—such as lactose intolerance and gastrointestinal disorders—or eating the same foods that cause belching. In addition, bloating can signal water retention—medically known as *edema*—from eating too many salty foods or taking certain drugs, especially birth control or other estrogen-containing pills. Edema can also be a telltale sign of hypertension and hormonal changes related to menstruation and pregnancy.

SIGNIFICANT FACT

About 70% of African Americans are lactose-intolerant. Asians and Jews are also at increased risk.

Being bloated can also be a sign of a variety of intestinal problems, including constipation, bowel obstruction, irritable bowel syndrome, and cancers of the digestive system, such as colon and stomach cancer. It can also signal thyroid disease, cirrhosis of the liver, and chronic kidney disease.

Bloating can also be an early—and sometimes the only—warning sign of *ovarian cancer,* the deadliest and one of the most underdiagnosed cancers in women. The prognosis is good if diagnosed early. Unfortunately, most cases—80%—aren't caught early enough to save a woman's life.

WARNING SIGN

The signs of ovarian cancer are so vague they're often ignored or confused with other, less serious conditions.

In June 2007, the American Cancer Society and other medical associations officially recognized the following as early warning signs of ovarian cancer, particularly if they last for more than just a few weeks:

- Pelvic or abdominal pain
- Difficulty eating or feeling full quickly
- Feeling a frequent or urgent need to urinate

THE SCOOP ON POOP

A variety of terms are used to describe the solid waste our bodies produce. There are formal ones, such as *bowel movement (BM), feces, excrement,* and *stool,* and more colloquial ones, including *poop, poo, caca, crap, doody, doo-doo, dump,* and *turd.* And then there's arguably the most popular but least socially acceptable word, *shit.*

Regardless of what it's called, most of us don't like to talk about it, much less look at or smell it. However, by observing if our stools float, sink, or stink, for example, we can learn a heap of information about our health. These qualities, as well as the color, texture, size, shape, and quantity of our poop, are affected by many factors, not the least of which is our diet. The saying "What goes in one end comes out the other" is totally true when it comes to waste products. But other elements come into play, too, all of which can affect the way your stools look as well as your bowel habits.

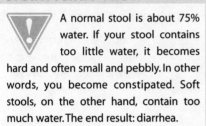

SIGNIFICANT FACT

A normal stool is about 75% water. If your stool contains too little water, it becomes hard and often small and pebbly. In other words, you become constipated. Soft stools, on the other hand, contain too much water. The end result: diarrhea.

Next time you're on the john, rather than burying your head in the tabloids to get the latest dirt on Hollywood stars, you may be better off getting the scoop on your own poop. You may lift the lid on a myriad of medical conditions, some of which may even be life-threatening.

GREEN STOOLS

A green planet is something most of us would love to have, but green stools? In fact, green stools may be a perfectly healthy and benign sign that you've been eating a lot of green vegetables, which are rich in chlorophyll (the green pigment in plants). Or they might mean you've been pigging out on lime Jell-O or too many green bagels and cupcakes on St. Patrick's Day.

Green stools are also a common result of taking iron supplements and certain antibiotics. Along with

SIGN OF THE TIMES

Before modern plumbing, people often sat on wooden stools to defecate. The euphemism for defecating was "going to stool." By the 16th century, the word *stool* had become synonymous with *feces.* Interestingly, this term is used more commonly today in the practice of medicine than the more scientific ones *excrement* or *feces.*

loose stools, green stools can be a reaction to the overuse of laxatives or any other substance that causes diarrhea. And if you look a bit "green around the gills," too, your green, loose stools are probably an indication of a GI infection or other diarrhea-causing condition.

ORANGE STOOLS

Noticing that your stools are orange can be quite disquieting; you may worry that the color comes from blood. But the orange color may merely mean that you've been eating a lot of foods containing beta-carotene, an important antioxidant found in such orange-colored foods as carrots, mangoes, sweet potatoes, apricots, and pumpkins. Likewise, taking too many beta-carotene (vitamin A) supplements, or eating foods with orange or red dye, can have the same effect. Orange stools are also a common reaction to the drug *rifampin*, which is used to treat certain bacterial infections, especially tuberculosis. (See **Golden Pee**, below.)

SIGNIFICANT FACT

Bile, a greenish yellow digestive juice made by the liver and stored in the gallbladder, helps break down fat and get rid of body wastes. Normally, as the bile moves through the intestines, it mixes with bacteria and turns brown. The end result: brown poop.

RED OR MAROON STOOLS

We all see red occasionally. However, seeing red in your stools may set off a red alert. Fortunately, sometimes it's just a false alarm. While what you're seeing may indeed be blood and signal a serious disorder, it can also be a harmless sign that you've eaten or drunk large amounts of something red.

SIGN OF THE TIMES

It's not just leeches and maggots that have recently caught on for medical treatments. The eggs of intestinal worms found in pigs are worming their way into the treatment of inflammatory bowel disease. A University of Iowa gastroenterologist has been successfully treating IBD patients with soft drinks mixed with 2,000 whipworm eggs. The eggs help regulate the body's immune system as well as reduce the intestinal inflammation in people with IBD. In the past, when most people harbored these and other parasites, the incidence of IBD was much lower.

Beets, tomato juice, red gelatin, and red fruit punches and ice pops are all common culprits.

On the other hand, if you see bright red streaks or spots on your stool—medically known as *hematochezia*—or on your toilet paper or in the toilet bowl, it can be a tip-off that you have bleeding *hemorrhoids* or *anal fissures* (tears) or other rectal or anal injuries. These injuries can result from childbirth, constipation, anal intercourse, or the insertion of objects into the rectum.

In addition to being a sign of hemorrhoids and fissures, red stools can signal problems along the gastrointestinal (GI) tract. If the stools are bright red, it's likely to be a sign of a problem in the lower GI tract, especially the colon. Hematochezia can, for example, be a sign of *diverticulitis*, a condition that occurs when the small pouches in the colon become irritated or infected. There may also be pain or tenderness, often on the lower left side. If the stools are dark red, the problem is more likely to be in the upper tract, which includes the esophagus, stomach, and small intestine. (See **Black, Tarry Stools,** below.)

SIGNIFICANT FACT

Because they have similar names, *irritable bowel syndrome (IBS)* and *inflammatory bowel disease (IBD)* are often mistaken for each other.

- IBS is more common and involves a cluster of signs that typically includes abdominal discomfort or pain and alternating bouts of diarrhea and constipation.
- IBD is much rarer and usually more serious and refers to two chronic diseases, *Crohn's* and *ulcerative colitis*. IBD can cause severe cramping, diarrhea, and bloody stools.

WARNING SIGN

A bloody stool is often the only warning sign of a colon polyp, which can become cancerous, or even colon cancer itself.

Bloody-looking stools may also signal an intestinal infection or even the presence of parasites. In addition, red stools can be a sign of IBD. (See **Frequent Farting,** above.) Other IBD signs may include diarrhea, cramps, nausea, and weight loss, among others.

Reddish stools may also be a reaction to certain medications, including potassium pills and some antibiotics, which can cause bowel ulcerations and subsequent bleeding. Lastly, red stools are often a red flag for colon polyps or colon cancer. The bottom line is that anything that causes bleeding in the GI system, from the mouth to the anus, can result in reddish or bloody stools.

BLACK, TARRY STOOLS

Black stools may seem even more sinister than red stools. But, in fact, they can be quite benign and merely a sign that you've been taking iron supplements, charcoal (to control gas), or Pepto-Bismol or other medicines containing bismuth. Black licorice (the real kind) as well as blueberries can also turn your stool black.

But if your poop is black and tarry—medically known as *melena*—it can signal the presence of blood. When blood travels from the upper GI tract (usually the esophagus or stomach) to the lower tract (the intestines and rectum), it becomes sticky and stinky.

WARNING SIGNS

If persistent, the following can be warning signs of colon cancer or another serious problem:

- Change in bowel habits
- Obvious blood in the stool
- Very dark-colored stool
- Pencil-thin stools
- Diarrhea or constipation
- A feeling that the bowel doesn't empty completely
- Unexplainable weight loss
- Excessive fatigue
- Vomiting

Black, tarry stools are also a common sign of a bleeding ulcer in the stomach (aka *gastric* or *peptic ulcer*) or *duodenum* (part of the small intestine). In addition, they can be a sign of alcohol abuse, as well as of the chronic use of certain drugs that can cause the stomach to bleed. The common culprits include aspirin, ibuprofen, naproxen, and other non-steroidal anti-inflammatory drugs (NSAIDs), as well as acetaminophen. Melena can also signal *gastritis,* an inflammation of the stomach lining, or cancer anywhere in the upper GI tract.

PALE POOP

You may think the importance of pale poop pales by comparison to that of black or red poop, and in some cases you may be right. Occasional pale, yellow, or even light gray poop can be a sign of having eaten a lot of white or light-colored food such as rice, potatoes, or tapioca. People who've had barium X-rays may notice that they have chalk-colored stools for a few days afterward. Antacids, calcium supplements, and some antidiarrhea drugs can have the same effect.

On the other hand, persistently pale poop—medically known as *acholic stool*—can be a tip-off that bile is not reaching the intestines. The blockage can be a sign of a tumor in the bile duct or the pancreas. Acholic stool can signal a number of serious liver diseases that involve blocked bile ducts, such as hepatitis, cirrhosis, and liver cancer. Other possible signs of a blocked bile duct include dark yellow or brown urine (see **Tea-Colored Pee,** below), yellow (jaundiced) eyes and skin, itching, and occasional pain.

SIGN OF THE TIMES

A common type of German toilet, the *Flachspueler,* literally meaning "flat flushing," is designed to facilitate stool studying. The toilet's flat surface catches the poop before it plops into the bowl. One downside is that it may take many flushes to wipe the surface clean. Another is the splash that can occur from peeing standing up. To spare the seat and standers from being spritzed, men are strongly urged to sit while peeing. To help enforce this *"Sitzpinkel* rule," this little sticker can be found under the lids of many toilets:

FLOATING FECES

Have you ever had to flush the toilet again and again, to no avail? Most of the time, stools sink, but sometimes the poop persistently pops to the surface. It used to be believed that fat was responsible for these "floaters," as they're commonly called. But it's actually excess gas that's keeping the feces afloat. If the gas is caused by your diet, the floaters are nothing to worry about—that is, unless someone is going to use the bathroom immediately after you.

HEALTHY SIGN

The average healthy stool has the consistency of a ripe banana, the shape of a sausage, and the color of a hamburger.

On the other hand, if the gas is the result of a GI disorder, the floaters can signal *celiac disease* (aka *sprue*, a condition in which a person cannot digest gluten, which is found predominantly in wheat). Floating stools are also seen with IBS or IBD. (See **Frequent Farting**, above.) People with these GI problems often have diarrhea along with the floating feces.

GREASY, SMELLY STOOLS

If you notice your floating stools have an oily coating and are frothy and foul-smelling, you have the classic signs of *steatorrhea*, an abnormally high level of fat in the stool. These fatty, fetid feces can be a sign of IBD (see **Red or Maroon Stools,** above) or may mean that your diet is too rich in fat and/or that your body isn't properly absorbing fat. Indeed, persistent steatorrhea often signals *malabsorption syndrome,* a condition in which fat and other nutrients aren't adequately absorbed in the digestive tract.

SIGNIFICANT FACT

Many people believe that if they don't have a bowel movement every day, it's a sign of constipation. But for some, it's perfectly normal not to have one for several days in a row. Constipation is actually defined as having fewer than three bowel movements a week and/or having small, dry, hard stools that are difficult to pass.

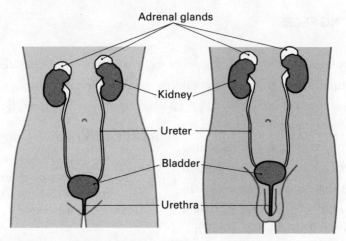

Adrenal glands

Kidney

Ureter

Bladder

Urethra

FEMALE AND MALE URINARY TRACT ANATOMY

Because the excess fat may be due to a blocked bile duct, steatorrhea can sometimes signal many of the same conditions as pale stools: gallbladder, liver, or pancreatic diseases, or cancer. (See **Pale Poop,** above.)

SLIMY STOOLS

If your stools look more like they're covered with mucus or pus than fat, it can be a sign of food allergies. And, as with fatty stools, they can also indicate GI tract problems such as bacterial infections, bowel obstructions, IBS, and IBD. (See **Red or Maroon Stools,** above).

Slimy stools sometimes signal the intestinal bacterial infection *shigellosis* or the parasitic infection *giardiasis.* Finally, mucus in the stool can be a telltale sign of rectal problems such as *proctitis,* an inflammation of the lining of the rectum.

SKINNY STOOLS

Skinniness isn't always a desirable state. If you've noticed that your stools have become narrow or ribbon-like, it's not a good sign. It can signal IBS, IBD (see **Floating Feces,** and **Red or Maroon Stools,** above), or a partial bowel obstruction—possibly from an adhesion, polyp, tumor, or cancer. Indeed, pencil-thin stools are an important early warning sign of colon cancer.

YOUR URINE

Our mothers likely spent many weeks, months, or in some cases even years potty-training us. Aside from the occasional childhood and adolescent fascination with bathroom jokes, once we've mastered control of the bladder, we rarely give peeing a second thought. We may not need to go as far as physicians in the Middle Ages, who obsessively inspected their patients' urine with such reverence, they might have been liquid gold. But we can learn a great deal about the state of our health by paying attention to what flows out of our bodies.

> **SIGNIFICANT FACT**
>
> Our internal plumbing system cleans about 200 quarts of body fluid every day. All but 2 quarts are returned squeaky clean into our circulatory system. The remainder is flushed out when we urinate.

Like defecation, urination goes by a wide variety of names, both naughty and nice. Whether you call it by the more socially acceptable terms (*micturition, urination, voiding*) or the more popular and colorful terms (*peeing, pissing, tinkling, taking a whiz,* or *taking a leak*), it's a good idea to take a peek at your pee now and then.

COLORED URINE

We might enjoy being tickled pink, but if we tinkle pink, it's another story—one that may not be something to giggle about. While urine that's pink, orange, green, or tea-colored may merely mean that you've been eating foods or taking medicines that contain coloring, sometimes the rainbow of hues in your urine can give you valuable clues to possible plumbing and pumping problems, infections, and even damage to your internal organs.

Pea-Green Pee

Like many urine-color changes, peeing green may be the end product of green-colored food or drink. Asparagus is a common culprit, which—as many of us are aware—can also make your pee smell funny. (See **Smelly Urine,** below.) And green pee is a fairly common reaction to certain multivitamins and some drugs used to treat depression, allergies, nausea, pain, and inflammation. Patients who've been given the anesthetic propofol sometimes pee green after surgery (although some have been known to pee pink).

But green urine can also be evidence of a buildup of bilirubin, the greenish chemical found in bile and produced by the liver that's also responsible for jaundice. (See Chapter 2.) Excess bilirubin may signal diseases of the liver and pancreas. (See **Pale Poop,** above.)

Pink or Reddish Pee

Pink or red urine doesn't always mean blood. Foods rich in red pigments, such as beets, red peppers, and blackberries, can turn the urine a rosy hue. Beet-red urine—medically called *beeturia*—is also often seen when people who are iron-deficient or have a malabsorption syndrome, eat beets (or sometimes other red foods). (See **Greasy, Smelly Stools,** above.)

Rhubarb and senna may turn your pee pink, too. They contain anthraquinone, which is often used as a dye and is a potent laxative. Pink or reddish urine can also be a reaction to several psychiatric drugs, as well as anthraquinone-containing anticancer agents.

Unfortunately, pink or reddish pee does sometimes signal blood in the urine—medically known as *hematuria.* It can, for example, be a sign of an injury to the kidney. But the blood can originate anywhere along the urinary tract. It can be an important early warning sign of several serious kidney, liver, or bladder conditions, including infections, stones, cysts, tumors, and even cancer.

Purplish Pee

Dark red or purplish urine is the hallmark of a rare group of usually inherited blood disorders called *porphyrias.* These disorders are very common in some European royal families but are not restricted to the blue bloods (so to speak) among us.

Interestingly, the urine may not turn purple until it's exposed to light for a while. Porphyrias produce many body signs, which range from light sensitivity and rashes to severe abdominal pain, mental confusion, epileptic seizures, and even paralysis.

SIGN OF THE TIMES

Several members of the British royal family suffered from porphyria. Mary, Queen of Scots, and her son King James I of England had the disease. George III had such a severe case that he became progressively insane and blind. His suffering was graphically depicted in the 1994 British film *The Madness of King George.*

Golden Pee

Our urine should be clear or have only a slight yellow hue. Dark yellow to orange urine can be an alert that you're seriously dehydrated. Off-smelling urine is another unmistakable sign of dehydration. (See **Tea-Colored Pee** and **Smelly Urine,** below.) Scanty urine—medically known as *oliguria*—is another important clue to dehydration.

SIGNIFICANT FACT

In Western cultures, the average person produces almost half a pound of feces a day.

Dark yellow urine may signal that you're taking in large amounts of beta-carotene from either foods or supplements. Some drugs will turn urine a true orange. High on the list are the antituberculosis drug rifampin, the blood thinner warfarin, and some cancer drugs. These are many of the same medications that turn stools orange. (See **Orange Stools,** above.)

Tea-Colored Pee

You shouldn't have to be a reader of tea leaves to know that dark, tea-colored urine can be a portentous sign of several significant conditions.

SIGN OF THE TIMES

Rhabdomyolysis was first reported in 1881 in the German medical literature. But it wasn't until the blitz of London in 1941 that it was identified as the major complication of people crushed under falling buildings and bridges.

Urine that looks like strong tea is another important sign of dehydration. Or, as with other colored urine, it may merely be a reaction to certain foods and medicines. For example, rhubarb can turn the urine very dark, as well as pink or red. (See **Pink or Reddish Pee**, above.) Quinine can cause tea-colored pee, too. It's found in drinks or in drugs, as well as some antibiotics, especially metronidazole (Flagyl), which is commonly used to treat certain intestinal infections, such as *giardiasis* and *dysentery*, and the vaginal infection *trichomonas*.

SIGN OF THE TIMES

Our ancestors found lots of uses for urine. Ancient Romans used it to clean their clothes and whiten their teeth. Portuguese urine was especially prized for this purpose. The ancient Chinese used urine as a mouthwash. On battlefields, both ancient and modern, it's been used to sterilize wounds when antiseptics were unavailable. And throughout history, people have drunk it in an attempt to cure their ailments.

Pee that looks like tea is also a sign of several serious medical conditions, including bleeding from the kidney or bladder that has stopped, allowing the blood in the urine to turn brown, as well as the liver diseases *hepatitis* and *cirrhosis*. Jaundice of the eyes, skin, and stools is another color-related body sign of liver disease. (See Chapters 2 and 9 and **Pale Poop**, above.)

Tea-colored urine can also signal *diabetic ketoacidosis (DKA)*, a life-threatening complication of diabetes. (See **Frequent Urination**, and **Sweet Pee**, below.) Finally, tea-colored urine is usually the first sign of *rhabdomyolysis*, a potentially fatal disorder in which skeletal muscle fibers break down, become toxic, and leak into the bloodstream. It's often the result of what's called a "crush injury"—the type of severe muscle damage you can get after being pinned in a car crash or crushed by a heavy object. Alcoholics who've had severe *delirium tremens (DTs)* can also have this condition.

HEALTHY SIGN

You might think that urine is supposed to be yellow, but it's really not. Healthy urine is clear or slightly yellow, and not foamy or frothy.

Overexertion from such activities as marathon running or strenuous bodybuilding can also lead to this disorder. In essence, rhabdomyolysis can result from any injury, disease, or disorder that causes skeletal muscle destruction. The encouraging news is that this condition is treatable when caught early; but if not, nerve or muscle damage, kidney failure, and potentially fatal blood clotting disorders and heart arrhythmias can occur.

SIGN OF THE TIMES

Self-conscious users of Japanese public toilets can mask the sound of their farts and other bodily functions with the simple push of a button. The toilets have devices that simulate the sound of a flushing toilet.

WARNING SIGN

If you're on certain cholesterol-lowering medicines, watch out for tea-colored urine, as well as stiff, achy, or weak muscles. These can be signs of *rhabdomyolysis*, a serious side effect.

SMELLY URINE

Some of our favorite foods (and some of our least favorites) can make our urine downright stinky. Asparagus, cabbage, cauliflower, and garlic can all produce malodorous urine. But some distinct or disagreeable urine odors can also alert you to medical problems. While it may not be too unusual to smell ammonia in the "john," if your urine smells like this cleaning agent, it can be a sign that you're dehydrated. (See **Golden Pee,** above.)

Also, foul-smelling urine—particularly the first pee of the day—may be a sign of a *urinary tract infection (UTI)*. (See **Cloudy Urine,** below.)

Fishy-smelling pee can signal a metabolic disorder graphically known as *fish odor syndrome* or by the more unpronounceable term *trimethyl-aminuria*. (See **Fishy-Smelling Sweat,** below.)

SWEET PEE

For many of us, spritzing and spraying with perfumes and eau de toilette is part of our daily bathroom ritual. But if the "eau" in your toilet is sweet-smelling, it's not a good sign. Indeed, it can signal a serious complication of diabetes known as *diabetic ketoacidosis (DKA)*. In DKA, substances called *ketones* can build up in the blood and give the urine, breath, and even skin a distinct sweet or acetone-like smell. (See **Smelly Sweat,** below.) Dark-colored urine (see **Tea-Colored Pee,** above) and excessive urination are other urine-related signs of this condition. Without treatment, DKA can lead to heart attacks, kidney failure, coma, and death.

FOAMY URINE

If you look down in the bowl and see bubbly urine, don't assume that the toilet's just been cleaned and some soap residue's been left behind. Foamy urine can be the very first sign of *proteinuria* (sometimes called *al-buminuria*), a buildup of bile salts or the protein albumin in the urine.

Proteinuria is a marker of kidney damage and heart disease, particularly in patients who have diabetes or hypertension. Foamy urine is also often the first sign of *nephrotic syndrome,* a serious dis-

> **SIGN OF THE TIMES**
>
>
> In ancient times, physicians would taste a patient's urine as a part of diagnosis. If it was sweet, they knew something was wrong. Sweet urine is now a recognized sign of diabetes. In fact, the term *diabetes mellitus* comes from the Greek word *diabetes*, "to flow," and the Latin word *mellitus*, "honey."

order in which the kidneys' filtering system can be damaged from viral infections, diabetes, and lupus. (See Appendix I.) This causes excess protein to find its way into the urine. Bubbles in the urine can also be a sign of a *fistula,* an abnormal connection between the bladder and the vagina or rectum. Any number of conditions, including Crohn's disease (see **A Gurgling Stomach,** above) or a tumor, can cause a fistula.

CLOUDY URINE

Murky or cloudy *(turbid)* urine is the hallmark of a UTI. Sometimes the urine will smell foul, too. (See **Smelly Urine,** above.) The infection can start and stay in the bladder, in which case it's medically known as *cystitis,* or it can move up the line and infect the kidneys, a condition called *pyelonephritis.* The cloudiness is due to bacteria and mucus in the urine. Infections can be found in other portions of the urinary tract, such as the urethra and ureters, and are often linked to sexual activity.

In men, cloudy or reddish-tinted urine can be a sign of an inflammation of the prostate, medically known as *prostatitis,* which is usually the result of a UTI, or sometimes an STD. Men with enlarged prostates, medically known as *benign prostatic hyperplasia* (**BPH**), are more susceptible to prostatitis, usually from a UTI. (See **Frequent Urination,** below.) In BPH, which is common as men age, the growing prostate gland blocks urine flow. Other urinary signs of prostatitis—whatever the cause—include difficulty urinating, a burning sensation or dribbling when urinating, and feeling like you haven't emptied your bladder completely. It's unclear whether there's any connection between prostatitis and prostate cancer.

HEALTHY SIGN

 In a healthy person, urine is virtually sterile and nearly odorless when it leaves the body.

In women, a UTI can be a sign of frequent or sometimes overly vigorous sexual activity. During sex, bacteria can be pushed up the urethra, the conduit for urine's exit out of the bladder and body. Women have relatively short urethras, which allow bacteria to get into the bladder quickly. Men, on the other hand, have longer urethras, which may be why UTIs are more common in women than men. But men with BPH (see

Frequent Urination, below) are at increased risk because they often are unable to completely empty their bladders. The remaining urine is fertile ground in which bacteria can grow. People with diabetes and those whose immune systems are compromised are also particularly vulnerable to UTIs.

WARNING SIGNS

Here are the common urinary-related signs of a UTI:
- A burning feeling when urinating
- Feeling like you need to urinate more than usual
- Feeling like you need to urinate but not being able to or only going a little
- Leaking urine
- Smelly, cloudy, dark, bloody urine

If you've had one bout of a UTI, you're likely to get another. Unfortunately, frequent attacks can be an early warning that you may be headed for trouble up the urinary tract in the kidneys. And kidney infections can cause permanent damage.

WARNING SIGN

Waiting too long to pee after you get the urge raises the chances of getting a UTI. A very full bladder will stretch and weaken the muscles that control voiding, causing incomplete emptying. Old urine left in the bladder is a fertile site for bacteria to grow.

FREQUENT URINATION

What can be more annoying and embarrassing than going to the theater and realizing you won't make it through the first act without going to the restroom? Or, even worse, you're an actor onstage or a speaker at the podium and desperately have to pee in the middle of your speech, even though you went before going on. If this happens with great frequency, you have the classic sign of what's aptly called *urinary frequency* or *polyuria.*

This is one of the most typical signs of pregnancy. But even if you're pregnant, it's not something that you should ignore (not that you could). Frequent urination—in men as well as women—particularly when teamed with thirst, is a very common and important early warning sign of diabetes. (See Appendix I.)

Polyuria may also signal a UTI or an STD. (See **Cloudy Urine,** above.) With both conditions, you may have a discharge as well. (See **Penile Discharge** and **Vaginal Discharge,** above.)

In older women, urinating more often than before is an all-too-common sign of menopause. As estrogen levels wane, the lining of the urethra thins and the surrounding pelvic muscle weakens. This leads not only to frequent urination but also to other *genitourinary* problems such as vaginal yeast infections and UTIs. (See **Penile Discharge** and **Vaginal Discharge,** above.)

But if you're an older man and have to pee a lot, it can be one of the classic signs of BPH. (See **Cloudy Urine,** above.) In BPH, an enlargement of the prostate (the walnut-sized gland that sits below the bladder and surrounds the ure-thra) compresses the urethra and blocks urine flow. As a result, the bladder can't empty quickly or completely, and the man feels the need to pee more often.

SIGN OF THE TIMES

It may not be everyone's cup of tea, but some well-known people have subscribed to the "urine cure"—a practice called *urophagia.* Gandhi, Jim Morrison, and Steve McQueen were purported to have drunk urine to relieve what ailed them.

SIGN OF THE TIMES

Because UTI is often linked to increased sexual activity, it used to be known by the naive and anachronistic term "honeymoon cystitis."

WARNING SIGNS

The following are typical urinary signs of BPH:
- Frequently urinating
- An urgent need to urinate
- A slow start
- Dribbling even after you think you've finished
- Feeling like your bladder isn't completely empty after you pee

BPH usually develops slowly as men age; in fact, nearly 90% of men will have this condition by the time they reach their 80s. As its name implies, BPH is not at all dangerous—except to a man's quality of life.

While constantly running to the "john" all day is a nuisance, jumping out of bed several times a night to pee is even more so. Having to urinate a lot at night—medically known as *nocturia*—can be a wake-up call, alerting you to several benign or not-so-benign conditions. It may, for example, be the result of an undesirable reaction to some common drugs, including diuretics, heart medications, and some psychiatric medications. And it can, of course, be a sign of the same conditions that cause frequent urination during the day, such as diabetes and BPH. Nocturia can also signal kidney disease and even heart failure. Or, not surprisingly, it can be a sign that you're drinking too many liquids, especially caffeinated drinks, beer, or other alcoholic beverages.

SIGNIFICANT FACTS

Any part of the urinary tract, upper or lower, can be home to a UTI.

- Kidneys: organs that make the urine
- Ureters: long tubes leading from the kidneys to the bladder
- Bladder: organ that stores the urine
- Urethra: tube through which urine leaves the bladder

LEAKING URINE

Most of us have probably laughed so hard at a good joke we've peed in our pants. But for about 13 million Americans who have *urinary incontinence,* peeing in their pants is no laughing matter. They suffer not only from this condition but also from the enormous social embarrassment that often follows. This can be especially troublesome for the elderly, who are at risk for this condition. But urinary incontinence is not just a problem of the elderly. About 30% of women and 5% of men between the ages of 15 and 64 have occasional leaking accidents.

HEALTHY SIGN

The average person urinates seven times a day—more or less can signal trouble.

Not all leaking problems are the same. For example, if a little pee drips out when you cough, sneeze, laugh, or exert yourself, it may be a sign of *stress incontinence*. In this condition, the muscles under the bladder can't hold up to the stress of the bladder filling up with urine for any one of a number of reasons. For example, the urethra doesn't close properly. As a result, even slight pressure on the bladder can squeeze out some pee.

Stress incontinence is the most common urinary leakage problem in young and middle-aged women, particularly in pregnant women. It's also frequently seen after childbirth or pelvic surgery, especially hysterectomy. It's a common sign of menopause, too. The fall in estrogen levels causes a drop in the urethra's ability to resist the flow of urine; the result is small amounts of urine trickling out. But men aren't immune to stress incontinence. It's often an unfortunate complication of prostate surgery.

For some people, just hearing the sound of running water can send them running to the toilet—sometimes not fast enough. This is an embarrassing sign of *urge incontinence* or *overactive bladder (OAB)*, a condition that causes people to become supersensitive to certain sounds and other signals that stimulate the bladder to start emptying, even if not full. Graphically known as *key-in-the-lock* or *garage-door syndrome*, OAB

SIGN OF THE TIMES

Approximately half of nursing home residents older than 65 years are incontinent. In fact, incontinence is often a major factor in the decision to place an elderly person in a nursing home.

SIGN OF THE TIMES

Not all urine is a waste.
- Urine is tested to help pinpoint ovulation.
- Urine is tested to confirm pregnancy.
- The urine of post-menopausal women has been collected for its abundance of the substances used in fertility treatment.
- The urine of pregnant women has also been collected to make fertility drugs.
- Last but not least, urine from pregnant horses has been a source of estrogens used in hormone replacement therapy in post-menopausal women.

affects more women than men, especially women under the age of 60, causing them to go to the bathroom frequently and even wet the bed at night *(nocturnal enuresis)*.

OAB can be a reaction to some drugs, especially diuretics, as well as caffeine-containing beverages, sedatives, and alcohol, all of which can act like diuretics.

SIGNIFICANT FACT

Leaking urine is common after childbirth. About 15% of women will still be leaking urine 3 months after having a baby.

It can also signal several serious medical conditions, including UTIs (see **Cloudy Urine,** above), vaginal infections and STDs (see **Penile Discharge** and **Vaginal Discharge,** above), and prostate cancer. It can also be a complication of radiation therapy or prostate surgery. Lastly, an overactive bladder is a common sign of several chronic conditions, including kidney and heart problems, diabetes, Parkinson's disease, and multiple sclerosis.

STOP SIGN

One good way to help avoid unintentional voiding is to do Kegel exercises, which help strengthen the pelvic floor muscles that control the bladder. There's an added benefit to these exercises: women who do them say sex is better.

SWEAT

We all sweat. And it's a good thing we do. Perspiring—medically known as *hidrosis*—is usually a healthy, benign sign that our sweat glands are doing their job regulating the body's temperature. It's natural for us to sweat from heat and strenuous exercise. We also might break into a "cold sweat" or have sweaty palms when we're emotionally stressed or very frightened.

Both temperature-regulating and emotional sweat come from the *eccrine glands,* which start functioning at birth.

With the exception of the lips, nail beds, and some parts of the vagina and penis, eccrine glands are found all over our bodies. Most are on the palms of our hands, the soles of our feet, under our armpits, and to a lesser degree on our faces.

We have another kind of sweat that comes from the *apocrine glands,* which only kick in after puberty. These sweat glands are also found under the arms, as well as around the nipples, and on hairy places, such as the scalp and genital region. Unlike eccrine glands, which regulate body temperature, apocrine glands don't react to heat, but they do produce sweat in response to emotions as well as to hormones.

SIGNIFICANT FACT

A single bead of sweat the size of a pea can reduce the temperature of a quart of blood by 1 degree Fahrenheit.

While no one's quite sure why they do what they do, apocrine glands seem to be important for sexual attraction—or repulsion, in some cases. They're thought to be a type of scent gland that emits a substance similar to *pheremones,* which are keys to successful mating in the animal world.

How much you sweat depends on many factors, including what and how much you eat and drink, what drugs you take, your hormone levels, your physical and emotional states, and even your genes.

PROFUSE PERSPIRATION

Do you find yourself sporting tank tops when others are shivering in turtleneck sweaters? Year-round excessive sweating is the hallmark of *hyperhidrosis,* a sometimes hereditary condition that causes a person to produce much more sweat than needed to regulate body temperature.

Hyperhidrosis can be triggered by high outdoor temperatures, overheated rooms, spicy foods, hot drinks, caffeine, and alcohol, as well as several medications. (See **Night Sweats,** below.)

WARNING SIGN

You may think it's good to sweat a lot, especially in the gym, but excessive sweating can cause you to lose calcium. (Yet another reason to take calcium supplements.) Sweating also stresses the heart. So if you have cardiac problems or are elderly, don't overdo it.

Excessive sweating in older women is often a telltale sign of menopause, and the sweating is usually worse at night. (See **Night Sweats,** below.) These hot flashes—or hot flushes, as they're sometimes called—are due to a drop in estrogen.

Older men, too, occasionally experience hot flashes, usually because of low levels of testosterone—medically known as *hypogonadism* (aka *andropause* or *male menopause*).

DANGER SIGN

If you break out in a cold sweat and feel light-headed or have chest or stomach pains, seek immediate medical attention. You may be having a heart attack.

Sweating profusely sometimes signals diabetes-related low blood sugar (hypoglycemia), which is usually accompanied by shakiness, dizziness, weakness, and hunger. Excessive sweating, along with heat intolerance, is a very common sign of hyperthyroidism. (See Appendix I.) In addition, profuse sweating is one of the three classic signs of a type of adrenal tumor, *pheochromocytoma,* which produces excess adrenaline. The other two characteristic signs are palpitations and headaches. If untreated, pheochromocytomas can be life-threatening because they can raise blood pressure to dangerous levels. They can also be cancerous.

SIGNIFICANT FACTS

We have about 3 to 4 million eccrine glands in our bodies. The sweat they produce is 99% water. The remaining 1% contains small amounts of salt, ammonia, calcium, and other minerals. These electrolytes regulate the body's balance of fluid and temperature.

Regardless of its cause, profuse perspiration can lead to athlete's foot, jock itch, prickly heat, warts, and nail infections, to say nothing of social embarrassment.

NIGHT SWEATS

Have you ever awakened at night drenched in sweat? If you're a woman, you'll recognize these night sweats as the baptism of menopause.

Excessive sweating at night (aka *nocturnal hyperhidrosis*) can be a sign of the same disorders as heavy sweating during the day (see **Profuse Perspiration,** above), but it may be more disturbing because it can severely disrupt sleep—both one's own and one's partner's.

Night sweats, as well as day sweats, are common reactions to many drugs. These include antihypertensives, antidepressants and other psychiatric drugs, cortisone, insulin, hormones, leuprolide (for infertility and prostate cancer), niacin (to lower cholesterol), tamoxifen (to treat breast and some other cancers), nitroglycerin (for angina), and some drugs for erectile dysfunction. Paradoxically, sweating at night is a common rebound reaction to antipyretic drugs—drugs such as aspirin, acetaminophen, ibuprofen, and other NSAIDs, which are used to lower fever. Night sweats can also signal anxiety, and unfortunately, some of the drugs used to treat anxiety can themselves cause night sweats. And night sweats can be a tip-off to alcohol and drug abuse.

In addition, sweating heavily at night can signal a number of systemic conditions, including GERD (see **Excessive Burping,** above), diabetes-related hypoglycemia, mononucleosis, and HIV/AIDS. Night sweats are also a classic clue to both *tuberculosis (TB)* and *malaria.* Cough and fever are other frequent signs of TB, while malaria is often accompanied by nausea, headaches, and chills. Interestingly, sweating often accompanies the chills that are also common with these infections.

Night sweats can be an early warning sign of some forms of cancer,

SIGNIFICANT FACT

Of the several million eccrine sweat glands distributed around our bodies, the hands and feet have the greatest concentration—about 3,000 per square inch. Only about 1% of the sweat our body produces comes from our armpits. Luckily, the sweat on our palms doesn't usually smell!

SIGNIFICANT FACT

Male sweat can be a turn-on to women, according to a recent study at the University of California, Berkeley. Male sweat contains the chemical androstenedione, which is sometimes added to perfumes and colognes as a potential aphrodisiac. Previously, male underarm sweat was shown to improve women's moods and even possibly affect ovulation. But this is the first study to show that a woman's hormones, sexual arousal, and mood are all affected by androstenedione.

especially *leukemia, Hodgkin's disease* (aka *Hodgkin's lymphoma*), and *non-Hodgkin's lymphoma.* These serious conditions often have other signs, such as weight loss and fever. But in the case of Hodgkin's, night sweats may be the only complaint.

SPEAKING OF SIGNS

The more you sweat in peacetime, the less you bleed during war.

—Chinese proverb

Finally, night sweats can be an early warning sign of a rare, slow-developing blood disorder, *poly-cythemia vera (PV),* a condition in which a person's bone marrow produces excess blood cells, especially red blood cells. Known by many other names, including *primary polycythemia, myeloproliferative disorder, Vasquez's disease,* and *Osler's disease,* it primarily affects people around the age of 60 and strikes more men than women. Other early signs of PV may include headaches, dizziness, itchiness after warm baths or showers, facial flushing, breathing difficulties, and a feeling of fullness in the up-

SPEAKING OF SIGNS

Horses sweat, men perspire, and women glow.

—Popular saying

per left abdomen. Some people experience vision problems, bleeding gums, and other bleeding problems. The extra red blood cells thicken the blood, possibly leading to tissue and organ damage as well as to strokes, heart attacks, or blood clots in the lungs, legs, and elsewhere. Indeed, without treatment, half the people with PV die within two years.

NO SWEAT

Some people never seem to sweat. No matter how hot and steamy it is, they remain cool as a cucumber. They may, in fact, have the hallmark of *hypohidrosis,* the decreased ability to sweat, or even *anhidrosis,* the inability to sweat. While you may think these conditions are enviable, you're wrong. They're potentially life-threatening because they can lead to hyperthermia, heat exhaustion, heat stroke, and ultimately death. The elderly are at especially high risk because they have a decreased ability to sweat anyway. They may not realize they're overheated until it's too late and they succumb to heat exhaustion.

Although sweat disorders can be signs of some serious genetic diseases, most cases are acquired. For example, hypohidrosis and anhidrosis—which can affect small or large areas of the body—can be a reaction to a number of medications, especially antihistamines or the drugs used to treat excessive sweating. A group of medications (called *anticholinergic agents*) used to treat high blood pressure and angina, psychiatric disorders, and muscle cramps can cause these sweat disorders as well.

In some cases diminished or nonexistent sweating can be evidence of damage to sweat glands from burns and other injuries, as well as various skin diseases. These sweating disorders can also signal some serious neurological disorders, such as Parkinson's disease and *Guillain-Barré syndrome* (see Chapter 7), an autoimmune nerve disorder that causes numbness, weakness, and sometimes paralysis of the limbs.

> ### SIGNIFICANT FACTS
>
> We all have a distinctive smell, which, like fingerprints, can theoretically be used to identify us, according to a recent study in Austria. The researchers also found that men and women have different sweat prints.

Lastly, little or no sweat may also signal *peripheral neuropathy,* which is common among diabetics (see Chapter 7) and *autonomic neuropathy,* a condition involving damage to the nerves that regulate sweating, heart rate, blood pressure, digestion, and other key body functions. Interestingly, autonomic neuropathy itself often signals diabetes. It can also be a clue to alcohol abuse, tumors, autoimmune disorders, and other serious diseases.

SMELLY SWEAT

Sweat itself doesn't smell. It's only when sweat mingles with bacteria, which are particularly abundant on the hairy areas of our bodies, that it gives off that distinctive stink. As anyone who's ever been in a gym realizes, body odor (aka BO) and sweat go hand in hand. The apocrine sweat glands are the prime culprits. (See **Sweat,** above.)

Not surprisingly, BO—medically known as *bromhidrosis*—is often strong evidence of poor personal hygiene or a disdain for deodorant. But smelly sweat can also be a clue to your culinary tastes. If you eat a lot of garlic or onions, or use curry or other strong spices, you might start smelling like your stockpot. This type of body odor is medically known as *eccrine bromhidrosis* because the odor emanates from the eccrine sweat glands. (See **Sweat,** above.)

SIGNIFICANT FACT

Americans spend almost $2 billion a year on deodorants and antiperspirants.

An odd odor can be a reaction to certain medications, including penicillin, some antidepressants, glaucoma drugs, and some cancer drugs. It can also be a strong hint that a person has been hitting the bottle too much. However, if someone's sweat smells like beer, it may not be from overindulging. Rather, it could signal a yeast infection. (See **Vaginal Discharge,** above.)

SIGN OF THE TIMES

In the past, many physicians sniffed out diseases by smelling their patients. Rubella smelled like plucked feathers, diphtheria had a sweet scent, typhoid smelled like freshly baked brown bread, and *scrofula* (tuberculosis of the lymph glands) gave off a stale beer smell.

Unpleasant or unusual body odors can also signal a number of other disorders. For example, if a person's sweat or urine smells sweet or like acetone, it might point to diabetes. (See **Sweet Pee,** above.)

Urine or Ammonia Body Odor

If someone smells of urine or ammonia, it can be a telltale sign that they've "had an accident," but it can also be a clue to kidney or liver disease. Ammonia-smelling sweat may also mean that a person is eating a protein-heavy diet. It may be evidence of infection with *Helicobacter pylori,* the bacterium responsible for some types of ulcers.

Fishy-Smelling Sweat

If your blind date smells fishy, it may merely mean he's a fishmonger. But it can reveal that he's into vitamin supplements and is taking a lot of choline, a type of B vitamin that helps metabolize fat. Or it might mean he has a liver disorder, which can prevent the breakdown of choline.

But fishy-smelling sweat could also signal a hereditary metabolic disorder aptly named *fish odor syndrome* (aka *trimethylaminuria*). People with this disorder can't metabolize trimethylamine, which is found in choline-rich foods such as eggs, liver, beef, and soy. Their urine and breath also emit a foul, fishy odor. (See Chapter 5 and **Smelly Urine,** above.) Although people with fish odor syndrome are generally physically healthy, they often suffer from social isolation and, as a result, depression.

SIGNING OFF

If you're experiencing abdominal or genital pain, have pain when urinating or defecating, or see blood in your stool or urine, see your doctor immediately. Also, if you have chronic or severe constipation or diarrhea or urinary incontinence, see your doctor as soon as possible for a diagnosis or referral to a specialist. If you're concerned about other below-the-belt signs or just have a gut feeling that something's wrong, don't hesitate to discuss it with your doctor. You might also want to consult or may be referred to one of the following specialists:

- *Endocrinologist:* A medical doctor who specializes in evaluating and treating hormone disorders.
- *Gastroenterologist:* A medical doctor who specializes in diseases and disorders of the gastrointestinal tract, including the esophagus, stomach, pancreas, and intestines.
- *Gynecologist:* A medical doctor who specializes in diagnosing and treating conditions related to the female reproductive system.
- *Proctologist:* A medical doctor who specializes in treating disorders of the rectum and anus.
- *Urologist:* A medical doctor who specializes in diagnosing and treating diseases and disorders of the urinary tract.

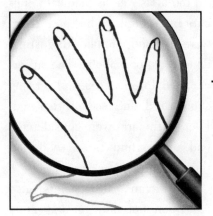

CHAPTER 9

SCRATCHING THE SURFACE

Your Skin and Nails

> The saying that beauty is but skin deep is but a skin-deep saying.
>
> —JOHN RUSKIN, 19TH-CENTURY ENGLISH WRITER AND CRITIC

Our skin—which, technically speaking, includes our hair and nails—is the largest of all our organs. (The liver is the second-largest.) Skin covers virtually every inch of our bodies, with the exception of our eyes and teeth. Our skin is also one of our most important organs; it's our living, breathing security blanket, and a waterproof one at that. Skin protects us from the assaults of our environment and provides a barrier to infections. It helps regulate our temperature, keeping us warm when it's cold and cool when it's hot. It also helps us maintain a healthy balance of fluids and minerals. And last but not least, our skin is the source of our sensory receptors for touch.

Skin is also the site of many, if not most, of our body signs. In fact, the majority of the signs we can see and touch are seen or felt on our skin, hair, or nails. And because they're so accessible, both to us and to others, skin signs can be as cosmetically disconcerting as they are diagnostically enlightening.

Since ancient times, people have been obsessed with skin diseases. In the Old Testament, for example, Leviticus 13 is taken up entirely with the diagnosis of leprosy and prevention of its spread by burning clothes and forced isolation.

Leprosy and other skin diseases had moral as well as medical implications—people who had them were deemed damned, disgusting, dangerous, or diabolic. The sufferers paid for their "sins" by being stigmatized and socially isolated. Even birthmarks were considered a bad omen, and those who had them were considered evil.

Physicians and others also read skin not only for indicators of evil but for signs of illness as well. Indeed, the reading of hands—known as palmistry or chiromancy—has been exceedingly popular for thousands of years in many cultures, and not just for reading the future. Aristotle and Galen read palms to assist them in diagnosing illness. By the Middle Ages, palm reading became identified with Gypsies and was banned by the Catholic Church as a form of devil worship.

Reading the hand's lines and lumps and bumps for accessing health and predicting the future still prevails today in parts of the Far East, not to mention the East Village in New York and much of the West Coast of the United States.

Nails, too, have had a key role to play throughout history, but more for their cosmetic importance than their medical significance. Our nails—which are also part of our skin—have been a focus of fashion

SIGN OF THE TIMES

Anthrax was first described in the Bible. The following cure was prescribed for the boils commonly caused by this disease: "Take a cluster of figs. And they took and laid it upon the boil, and he recovered."

In 2003, the National Institutes of Health and the pharmaceutical industry discussed the possibility of studying the use of fig plants as a treatment for anthrax.

SIGN OF THE TIMES

In the Middle Ages, you cursed your enemies by wishing a pox or some other skin disease on them. Or better still, you likened them to one; calling someone a "scurvy knave" was a favorite. Probably the worst skin-related insult was hurled by Shakespeare's King Lear at his daughter Goneril when he called her "a disease that's in my flesh...a boil, a plague-sore, an embossed carbuncle."

throughout the centuries. Today we still file, trim, clip, shape, buff, polish, and extend our nails, all with the intent to beautify and adorn them. However, the appearance of our nails reflects not only how meticulous (or even obsessed) we are with our appearance but also our medical history and nutritional status, not to mention, in many cases, our occupation.

A quick look at our nails can reveal reams about how well our bodies are working and possible diseases and disorders that may be lurking within. In fact, our finger- and toenails can be as informative about our health and well-being as our blood pressure or weight.

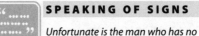

SPEAKING OF SIGNS

Unfortunate is the man who has no fingernails to scratch his head with.

—Arabian proverb

NAILING THE PROBLEM: YOUR NAILS

Our nails—or *nail plates,* as they are medically known—are composed primarily of the protein keratin. Although keratin is also found in our skin and hair, nails contain less water, so they're harder. Our nails' durability makes them ideal protectors of the blood vessels, nerves, and bones beneath.

Odd-colored or misshapen nails probably won't have you scratching at your doctor's door for attention. Luckily, however, most physicians take a peek at their patients' nails during office visits. Embedded in our nails are clues to a variety of medical disorders.

CHANGING NAIL COLORS

White Marks

We're probably all familiar with those occasional little white, irregular spots or lines scattered on our nails. These chalky marks—medically known as *leukonychia*—are usually benign signs of a minor injury to the nail, which normally disappear in time.

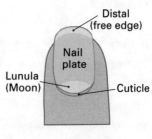

NAIL ANATOMY

White nail spots or marks can also be due to *onycholysis*. If you knew that, you've hit the nail on the head—both figuratively and possibly literally. Onycholysis is the separation of the nail from its nail bed. As anyone who's ever hit their own nail with a hammer knows, the nail will likely fall off.

HEALTHY SIGN

A healthy adult's nails grow at a constant, albeit slow, rate—about 1/8 of an inch a month. It takes 4 to 6 months for a totally new fingernail to grow. It takes 8 to 12 months for a new toenail to step in.

But sometimes white specks and stripes on, in, or under our nails aren't benign at all. These white marks can also signal such conditions as nail warts or fungus (*onychomycosis*) or such skin conditions as *psoriasis* and *eczema,* which can affect the nails. White nail spots can be one of the several signs of the systemic condition *sarcoidosis,* which affects the skin, lungs, and other organs. (See **Scaly Patches on the Face,** below, and Appendix I.) If the nail is soft in addition to having white spots—known as *Plummer's nails*—it can be a clue to hyperthyroidism. (See Appendix I.)

A Single White Line

A slightly thick white line going horizontally across the nail—called a *Mee's line*—is a classic sign of arsenic or thallium poisoning. But before you decide someone is trying to rub you out, think about this: Mee's lines can point to a wide variety of serious systemic conditions that can damage the nail, including *heart failure, Hodgkin's disease, malaria,* and even *leprosy.* Because these white lines, which tend to affect only one nail, are embedded in the nail itself, they will disappear when the nail grows out or if their underlying cause is successfully treated. In fact, this nail sign can help pinpoint when the illness (or poisoning) began. The lower down on the nail, the more recent the occurrence.

SIGNIFICANT FACT

As we age, our nails grow more slowly and may become dull, yellow, opaque, hard, brittle, and thick.

A Double White Line

If you notice two white horizontal narrow stripes on one or more nails, you have the classic sign of *Muehrcke's lines*. These lines are actually *in* the nail bed (the tissue under the hard nail), so they won't move or disappear as the nail grows. Muehrcke's lines are a very common sign of *hypoalbuminemia*, which is a lower-than-normal level of the protein albumin in the blood. Several acute and chronic medical conditions, including kidney disease, cirrhosis of the liver, heart failure, and malnutrition, among others, can produce this condition and these lines. However, most cases are due to an inflammatory response to an infection or injury.

SIGNIFICANT FACT

To tell the difference between Mee's lines and Muehrcke's lines, press on the white band. If the nail turns pink, it's a Muehrcke's line.

Two-Toned Nails

If half your nail is brown and the other half white—somewhat like New York City's famous black-and-white cookie—you may have what's aptly known as *half-and-half nails*. In this condition, the white part is at the cuticle end of the nail, while the brown part is nearer the tip. Unfortunately, half-and-half nails are common signs of chronic kidney disease.

SIGN OF THE TIMES

Farmers used to place a mark at the base of their thumbnail when they planted their land. When the little spot made its way to the nail tip, the farmers knew the little seeds had sprouted, grown into a plant, and were ready for harvest.

If, however, your nail is almost totally an opaque white color, you may have a form of leukonychia (see **White Marks,** above) called *Terry's nails*. With Terry's nails, which usually affect all your nails, the nails are whitish from the cuticle to almost the tip, at which point there's a dark pink or brown band. Sometimes the nails are so white and

TERRY'S NAILS

opaque that the moon of the nail—called the *lunula*—disappears. The white and brown colors are in the nail bed, not on the nail itself.

Terry's nails are a fairly common sign of aging. Unfortunately, and especially in younger people, these nails are often signs of cirrhosis of the liver, diabetes, chronic kidney failure, or congestive heart failure.

Blue Nails

While painting your nails blue may be a sign of youthful fancy or rebellion, naturally blue nails may be an important tip off that you're not getting enough oxygen—a condition medically known as *cyanosis*. As with blue lips, blue skin (See Chapter 5 and **Bluish Skin,** below), and other signs of cyanosis, blue nails can signal lung disease or *peripheral arterial disease* (PAD), among other circulatory problems. (See Chapter 7.) The nails of people with *Raynaud's disease,* which is considered a PAD, will sometimes turn blue, usually in response to cold or stress, then go back to normal once circulation returns. Blue nails can also signal a reaction to medications, such as antiviral drugs and the antibiotic tetracycline.

SPEAKING OF SIGNS

For three days after death, hair and fingernails continue to grow, but phone calls taper off.

—Johnny Carson, the late, late-night comedian

Yellow Nails

Yellowed nails may be a sign that someone's a heavy smoker or has taken the antibiotic tetracycline for some time. Or they may just be the telltale cosmetic clue of having used dark-colored nail polish, which can leave a yellow stain behind. But yellow nails can also signal something more serious.

Much like yellow eyes and skin (see Chapter 2 and **Yellowish Skin,** below), yellow nails can point to jaundice. They can also be a sign of AIDS. And yellow nails with a slight bluish base can signal diabetes.

But sometimes yellow nails—especially if they grow slowly, are very thick and curved, lose their cuticles, and even fall off—may signal a rare condition aptly named *yellow nail syndrome.* Besides having disfigured and yellowed nails, a person with yellow nail syndrome usually has a lung disease and/or *lymphedema,* a buildup of lymph fluid in the tissues. All the nails are usually affected and, unfortunately, nearly always permanently.

WARNING SIGN

Brownish, yellowish nails, sometimes with little white patches, can be signs of nail fungus. Your nails may smell bad, too.

Moon Color Changes

The pale, crescent-shaped area at the base of the nail is the nail moon, called the *lunula.* It can have as many colors as the celestial moon has phases. For example, a blue moon isn't just the name of an old song. Medically known as *azure lunula,* a blue nail moon can be a sign of *Wilson's disease,* an inherited degenerative liver disease in which there is a buildup of copper. A red nail moon, on the other hand, can

SIGNIFICANT FACT

Fingernails grow faster than toenails, and both grow faster in the summer than in winter. Nails on your dominant hand grow faster than those on your less-used hand. Lastly, men's nails grow faster than women's.

signal heart failure. And a yellow moon, like yellow nails (see **Yellow Nails,** above), can be a telltale sign that you've been taking the antibiotic tetracycline. Blue-gray moons can be warning signs of silver poisoning, and finally brown or black nail crescents may be pointing to an excess intake of fluoride.

STRANGE MARKINGS

Dark Stripes

Dark streaks can be evidence that you haven't heeded the warning to steer clear of undercooked pork or wild game and have acquired the parasitic disease *trichinosis.* Medically known as *splinter hemorrhages,*

HEALTHY SIGN

Healthy nails are:
- smooth
- slightly curved
- firm
- unblemished

these tiny horizontal stripes look like they're embedded in or just underneath the nail and are actually tiny hemorrhages in the nail bed. Splinter hemorrhages are also a classic sign of *endocarditis*, an infection of the heart. Or they can signal *vasculitis*, an inflammation of the blood vessels.

SIGNIFICANT FACTS

Aging slows nail growth. A totally new fingernail will take 3 months to grow in childhood but 6 months by the time we're 70.

Splinter hemorrhages may also point to several autoimmune diseases, including *psoriasis, lupus (SLE)* (see **Butterfly Mask,** below, and Appendix I), *rheumatoid arthritis,* and *antiphospholipid syndrome* (APS), a potentially serious blood clotting disorder. (See **Purplish Patches,** below.) Lastly, splinter hemorrhages can signal peptic ulcers and kidney disease.

SIGNIFICANT FACT

The acronym **ABCDEF** was devised to help draw attention to and diagnose *subungual melanoma.*

A: Age (most cases are seen in people age 40 to 60) and African Americans, Asians, and Native Americans

B: Brown to black band, a breadth of 3 mm or more, and variegated borders

C: Change in the color of the nail band that has appeared or no change in color after a treatment has been tried

D: Digit most commonly involved (the thumb and big toe)

E: Extension of the pigment onto the nail fold

F: Family or personal history of *dysplastic nevus* (an abnormal mole) or melanoma

Vertical Dark Bands

A dark, wide, longitudinal band on your nail—medically known as *melanonychia striata*—may occur as a reaction to tetracycline, antimalarial drugs, or some drugs used to treat cancer. When drugs are the cause, several nails are usually involved. The dark stripes can also signal a fungal infection, especially if this sign is seen on the toenail.

A dark stripe known as a *frictional melanonychia* on the toenail can be a tip-off that your shoes are too tight. If it's on a fingernail, you may be working a lot with your hands and injuring your nails. Benign dark, pigmented bands are common in people who are dark-skinned. In fact, more than three-quarters of black adults have one or more of them on their nails.

But whether you are fair- or dark-skinned, these brown or black bands shouldn't necessarily be taken lightly. This is especially true if the skin under the front of the nail (in particular a single nail) is also dark, or if the band runs into the nail fold on the side of the nail—medically called the *Hutchinson sign*. These can be ominous signs of *subungual melanoma*, a very dangerous type of skin cancer of the nail bed, which has a high rate of occurrence in certain racial groups, especially African Americans, Asians, and Native Americans. Unlike most other types of nail stripes, these don't disappear; rather, melanoma-associated streaks tend to grow. This type of skin cancer is found most often in people over age 50.

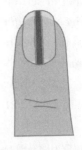

VERTICAL DARK BANDS
(Melanonychia Striata)

SIGNIFICANT FACT

 Half of the cases of melanoma in dark-skinned people occur as dark bands that run the length of the nail.

MISSHAPEN NAILS

Nails That Curve Downward

Nails with an exaggerated downward curve instead of just a slight slope—medically known as *clubbed nails*—aren't just un-sightly. The thickening of the *nail bed*, the soft tissue under the hard nail, causes the bulge. Unfortunately, nail clubbing usually develops so slowly that you may be unaware of its happening and, therefore, ignore this important sign. This type of change in nail shape is usually permanent.

Clubbed nails can point to a

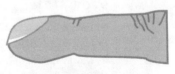

CLUBBED NAIL

SIGN OF THE TIMES

 In 2000, a retired photographer in India tried to auction off his world-record long nails to the highest bidder. Each nail was more than 3 feet long, and his longest was 4.8 feet! According to reports, they were thick, uneven, and looked like bumpy antlers or poorly crafted walking sticks. How he held a camera is unknown.

number of serious, even life-threatening conditions, including *cirrhois of the liver* and *inflammatory bowel disease*. (See Chapter 8.) They can also signal that your body isn't getting enough oxygen (*cyanosis*). In this case, the nails, as well as the skin, will probably take on a bluish tone. (See **Blue Nails**, above, and **Bluish Skin**, below.) And clubbed nails often go hand in hand with clubbed fingers (see Chapter 7), a common sign found in people with serious lung disease, including *chronic obstructive pulmonary disease* (*COPD*) and lung cancer.

Nails That Curve Upward

If the sides of your nails curl upward, commonly called *spooning*, it can signal a nutritional deficiency, such as of iron or vitamin B_{12}, which can cause anemia. And spooning—medically known as *koilonychia*—is a nail sign of such systemic disorders as Raynaud's disease (see Chapter 7 and **Blue Nails**, above) and lupus. (See **Butterfly Mask**, below and Appendix I.) It can also be a revealing sign that you've been exposed to petroleum-based products, possibly at work. If the fingernails are spooned and extremely thick, it can signal diabetes.

STOP SIGN

 To determine if a nail is spooned, perform the water drop test. Place a drop of water on the nail. If the drop does not slide off, then the nail is on its way to spooning.

TEXTURE TRANSFORMATIONS

Thick Nails

Thickening fingernails—medically called *onychauxis*—can be a benign sign of aging. Over time, however, they can become severely thickened and hook-like. When it affects the toenails, this nail deformity—medically called *onychogryposis* (aka *ram's horn nail*)—can make walking very difficult and particularly dangerous for older people. Thick nails can also signal an injury, infection, poor circulation, diabetes, or a poor diet.

WARNING SIGNS

The skin and nails of the hands can produce a wide variety of signs that point to diabetes:

- Thick, soft nails
- Beading (looks like tiny drips of candle wax)
- Spooned nails
- *Palmar xanthomas* (tiny fat deposits on the palms)
- Red palms

Rough Nails

Some people have rough nails with vertical ridges, medically known as *trachyonychia*. Because the nails also tend to look gray, opaque, and lackluster, they're commonly referred to as *sandpapered nails*. Trachyonychia can show up on any number of nails on the hands and feet. When all 20 nails are affected, it's aptly referred to as *20-nail dystrophy*.

Trachyonychia, which literally means "rough nails," is often seen in people with *lichen planus,* a fairly uncommon inflammatory disease of the skin and mouth that causes intense itching. (See Chapter 5.) Thin, splitting nails are also a sign of this condition. In fact, nail changes are sometimes the only sign of this disorder. In some cases of lichen planus, the nail undergoes *onycholysis*—separation of the nail from its bed—and in severe cases, the nail falls off and may never grow back.

Sandpapered nails can point to other skin and hair problems, including *psoriasis, eczema, vitiligo* (see **Large White Patches,** below), and *alopecia areata* (see Chapter 1). Unfortunately, even when the underlying problems are treated, the nail changes of trachyonychia are usually permanent.

Brittle Nails

For some of us, breaking a nail ranks right up there with a bad hair day. While many times we can chalk up brittle, cracked nails to dry weather and harsh cleaning solutions, they can also be clues to thyroid disease or a deficiency of iron or vitamin A. There's some debate whether calcium deficiency plays a role as well.

Pitted Nails

A small indentation on the nail, called *pitting*, can be a telltale sign of the common skin condition *psoriasis*. (See **Reddish Patches,** below.) In fact, up to half of psoriasis sufferers have these pinpoint depressions in their nails. But this nail deformity doesn't just occur with psoriasis. It's also a fairly common sign of several autoimmune disorders, including *Reiter's syndrome* (see **Scaly Rash on Palms or Soles,** below), which is a group of conditions that include joint, urinary, and eye problems; *sarcoidosis* (see **Scaly Patches on the Face,** below); *pemphigus,* which causes blistering and sores on skin and mucous membranes; and *alopecia areata,* which causes clumps of hair to fall out. (See Chapter 1.) Like many other problem nails, pitted nails may crumble and eventually fall off.

Horizontal Ridges

Grooves going from side to side on the nail—medically known as *Beau's lines*—can signal a wide variety of serious systemic conditions. These indentations look like little furrows dug into the nail. They may develop on one, several, or all nails. When more than one nail is affected, the lines usually show up on the identical spot on each nail.

Beau's lines are telltale signs that an illness or nail injury has tem-

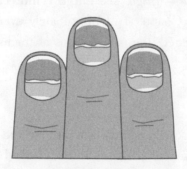

BEAU'S LINES

porarily halted nail growth. For example, Beau's lines are sometimes seen in people who've had a recent heart attack, surgery, infection, or cancer treatment. After treatment or recovery, the nails usually grow back normally.

These ridges sometimes occur on the nails of people with chronic conditions as well. They can, for example, signal Raynaud's disease (see **Blue Nails,** above, and Chapter 7) or *pemphigus* (see **Pitted Nails,** above).

WRAPPING IT ALL UP: YOUR SKIN

UNUSUAL SKIN COLORS

Pale Skin

Have you been told lately that you look as white as a ghost? If so, it shouldn't be taken lightly. Your pallor may be a sign of *anemia,* a condition in which there is a lower-than-normal amount of red blood cells. Although there are many types of anemia, the most common is *iron-deficiency anemia,* which is usually a sign of a diet too low in iron. While it is quite rare in men, fully 20% of women, and an astounding 50% of pregnant women, are iron-deficient.

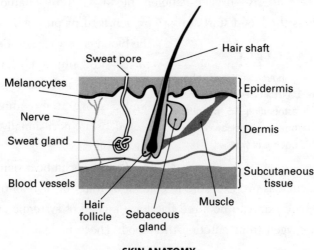

SKIN ANATOMY

Fatigue is another common sign of anemia, which is sometimes popularly referred to as "tired blood;" but other signs may include weakness, shortness of breath, irritability, and brittle nails. (See **Brittle Nails,** above.) The whites of the eyes (*sclera*) may also look blue.

SIGNIFICANT FACTS

- The skin is the largest organ of the body.
- The skin is the fastest-growing organ we have.
- There are approximately 19 million skin cells on every square inch of our bodies.

While most cases of anemia in women are diet-related or due to heavy menstrual bleeding, anemia in men and postmenopausal women often signals internal bleeding, especially from the gastrointestinal tract. The bleeding may come from ulcers or may be the result of overuse of aspirin and other nonsteroidal anti-inflammatory drugs (NSAIDs).

Anemia can be an early warning sign of leukemia as well as other cancers, particularly those of the stomach, colon, and esophagus. It often results from cancer treatments, too.

Bluish Skin

If you notice that your skin has recently taken on a bluish tinge, it may be a sign of *cyanosis*—oxygen-deficient blood. Well-oxygenated blood is bright red; as the blood starts to lose oxygen it turns purplish, and when

SIGNIFICANT FACT

Each hour, we shed about 600,000 particles of skin—that's an astounding 1.5 pounds a year. By age 70, the average person will have shed about 105 pounds of skin.

the blood is very oxygen-deprived it turns skin blue. The lips (see Chapter 5) and nails (see **Blue Nails,** above) are commonly affected, as are occasionally the feet, nose, and ears.

Cyanosis can be a sign of external factors such as overexposure to cold air or water or high altitudes. But persistent blue skin can be a red flag for a myriad of systemic conditions that block oxygen from entering the blood. These include lung diseases such as asthma, *chronic obstructive pulmonary disease* (COPD), and lung cancer. Cyanosis can also signal heart disease.

Yellowish Skin

If you notice a yellow cast to your skin, it's most likely the classic sign of *jaundice,* which also commonly causes the whites of the eyes to turn yellow. (See Chapter 2.) The yellow color comes from an excess of *bilirubin,* a yellow substance that is the normal by-product of the breakdown of red blood cells. But if your skin looks more orange than yellow, it may merely be a sign of *carotenemia* (see Chapter 7), a usually benign condition resulting from consuming too much beta-carotene or vitamin A, either from supplements or from foods such as carrots.

In some cases, yellow skin can be a sign of a hereditary, benign form of jaundice called *Gilbert's syndrome.* (See Chapter 2.) However, it's

WARNING SIGN

For some people the combination of wearing perfume or cologne and going out in the sun can cause skin discoloration, which can be permanent.

more likely to signal a liver disorder, such as hepatitis, cirrhosis, or liver cancer, or pancreatic cancer. Jaundice can also be a sign of hypothyroidism (see Appendix I) or *infectious mononucleosis,* a contagious viral infection also known as "the kissing disease."

WARNING SIGN

If your skin is excessively dry and you have dry, brittle hair and nails, it may signal hypothyroidism.

FACIAL MARKS AND MASKS

Rosy Cheeks

Does your face frequently flush or your cheeks get red, even when you're not embarrassed? If you're a woman, you may be having hot flashes, a classic sign of menopause. The redness of hot flashes usually vanishes quickly.

SIGNIFICANT FACTS

Each square inch of skin contains:
- 1,300 nerve cells
- 100 sweat glands
- 3 million cells
- 3 yards of blood vessels

If the flush persists, however, it may be an indication of *rosacea.* (See Chapter 4.) Rosacea is a type of rash that sometimes resembles a face mask or butterfly but is different from the "mask of lupus" (see **Butterfly Mask,** below) or the "mask of pregnancy" (see **Dark Patches on Cheeks,** below). In its early stages, rosacea may merely cause periodic flushing or blushing, but it then progresses to permanent redness on the face. The rosacea rash often consists of tiny pimples, which is why it's sometimes referred to as "adult acne," as well as small, dilated blood vessels just under the skin—medically known as *telangiectasia.* Some people develop rosacea on their torsos or limbs rather than on their faces. Other skin signs of rosacea may include itching and burning.

Rosacea is more common in women than men and tends to strike people between the ages of 30 and 40. It occurs most often in fair-skinned people, especially those of northern European or Celtic descent. Wind, sun, strenuous exercise, stress, spicy foods, and caffeine can all trigger or exacerbate rosacea. And it's especially common among people who abuse alcohol. In fact, alcohol-related rosacea is responsible for the bulbous noses often seen on heavy drinkers. (See Chapter 4.)

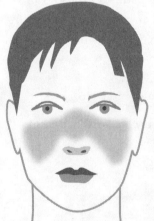

RASH OF ROSACEA

Facial flushing can also be the earliest sign of a very rare but very serious condition called *carcinoid syndrome,* which is caused by an uncommon type of cancer called *carcinoid tumor.* This type of tumor originates in the gastrointestinal tract and secretes large amounts of hormone-like substances, causing the blood vessels to dilate. Like the flushes from rosacea, carcinoid-syndrome-related flushes are often triggered by hot beverages, hot or spicy food, alcohol, and stress. However, the carcinoid flushes usually last for

HEALTHY SIGN

Healthy skin is:
- Smooth
- Supple
- Warm to the touch
- Cut-, scrape-, and bruise-free

only about 20 to 30 seconds and may be followed by a bluish tinge; the rosacea flushes persist for much longer. And unlike other types of flushes and blushes, during a carcinoid flush the face becomes beet red and is covered with the characteristic marks of telangiectasia.

Other signs of carcinoid syndrome may include shortness of breath, wheezing, cramps, and severe diarrhea. Unfortunately, by the time these signs appear, the cancer is usually quite advanced and has spread to the liver.

Butterfly Mask

A butterfly-shaped rash on the face—medically known as *malar erythema*—is the hallmark of *lupus*—medically known as *systemic lupus erythematosus* (SLE)—a very serious, chronic autoimmune inflammatory disease. (See Appendix I.) In fact, about half of people with SLE have this characteristic rash, which is referred to as "the butterfly rash of lupus" or the "mask of lupus." Like rosacea, lupus-related rashes are *photosensitive*—they can be triggered or worsened by sunlight. But unlike rosacea, these rashes are flat rather than bumpy.

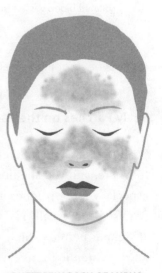

BUTTERFLY RASH OF LUPUS

Dark Patches on Cheeks

If you have dark symmetrical patches covering your cheeks and the bridge of your nose, like a face mask, you have the classic sign of *melasma* (aka *chloasma*), a type of hyperpigmentation. Melasma is much more common in women than men; dark-skinned women tend to develop this condition more than light-skinned women. Exposure to the sun and estrogen also increase the risk.

In a young woman, melasma is often a signal that she's pregnant. Indeed, it's so prevalent during pregnancy, affecting about half of pregnant women, usually during the second or third trimester, that it's often called the *mask of pregnancy*. The dark patches can also be a reaction to birth control pills or estrogen replacement therapy. The good news is that within months of stopping these medications or giving birth, the blotches fade.

> **SIGNIFICANT FACTS**
>
> Here are some useful skin definitions.
>
> - *Erythema:* unusual redness of the skin
> - *Macule:* flat spot that can be seen but not felt
> - *Melasma:* darkening of the skin
> - *Nevus* (pl. *nevi*): a mole, birthmark, or other mark on the skin
> - *Nodule:* solid bump under the skin
> - *Papule:* solid bump on the skin
> - *Pustule:* small, pus-filled bumps on the skin
> - *Telangiectasia:* visible, dilated blood vessels under the skin

Scaly Patches on the Face

Scaly patches of discolored skin smack in the middle of your face are hard to ignore, and you shouldn't. They may be telltale signs of *lupus pernio*, especially if the patches are persistent. Lupus pernio patches can be flat or raised and usually also appear on the cheek, nose, lips, and ears.

Lupus pernio (which shouldn't be confused with the more commonly known *systemic lupus erythematosus [SLE]*), is a chronic form of a fairly common inflammatory disease, *sarcoidosis* (see Appendix I), which produces tiny clumps of cells in various organs in your body. Sarcoidosis can affect not just the skin but also many other body organs, including the eyes, liver, lymph nodes, and lungs. In fact, the lungs are affected in 70% of the people with sarcoidosis, causing chronic coughing and shortness of breath. When the eyes are affected, dry eye, vision loss, glaucoma, and other eye problems can occur.

Sarcoidosis can produce other skin problems. When it affects the legs, ankles, or shins, it's called *erythema nodosum.*

Sarcoidosis often produces no signs at all. It's often discovered serendipitously; for example, when a person has an X-ray taken as part

SIGNIFICANT FACTS

Skin symptoms of sarcoidosis may include:
- Red rashes on the face and body
- Red lumps, particularly on the legs (erythema nodosum)
- Skin eruptions
- Purple patches
- Itching

of an examination before surgery or for another problem. When it does produce signs, however, skin signs are often the earliest ones, showing up on about one-third of people with this disease. Other early indicators of sarcoidosis may include fatigue, fever, chest pain, joint aches, and weight loss. These and other signs of sarcoidosis depend, in part, on the organ affected.

The course of this disease varies greatly among people: from mild to very serious, with or without flare-ups, and worsening or not. The signs can last a short time or for a year or more, or may even disappear. The good news is that in two-thirds of those with lung sarcoidosis, the disease improves or even spontaneously clears up.

SPEAKING OF SIGNS

I need sex for a clear complexion, but I'd rather do it for love.
—Actress Joan Crawford

Sarcoidosis is most typically found among people of Northern European and Scandinavian, especially Swedish, descent and African Americans; affects more women than men; and tends to strike people between the ages of 20 and 40. Interestingly, people of Swedish or European descent tend to have sarcoidis of the legs *(erythema nodosum),* while African American women are more likely to develop it on their face (lupus pernio).

BODY PATCHES AND PATTERNS

Large White Patches

Have you ever noticed someone with large white patches on their skin, reminiscent of the patches on a pinto pony? If so, they have the markings of *vitiligo* (also known as *leukoderma*), a skin condition that often runs in families and usually shows up before age 20.

SIGN OF THE TIMES

The term *vitiligo* was coined by the ancient Roman physician Celsus in the 2nd century A.D. The word itself is thought to derive from the Roman word for calf, *vitilus.* Calves often had white patches.

The white patches themselves are benign, but because they lack *melanin* (the substance that gives skin its color), they're highly susceptible to sunburn and, as a result, to skin cancer. (See **Reddish Patches,** below.)

Vitiligo can be a very early warning sign of autoimmune thyroid disease, especially Graves' disease, the most common type. (See Chapter 2.) In fact, about one-third of people with Graves' disease, as well as Hashimoto's thyroiditis (see Chapter 6), both of which also run in families, have these white patches. However, vitiligo may precede other signs of Graves' disease by several decades. People with vitiligo may also be at increased risk for various eye diseases.

SIGN OF THE TIMES

Michael Jackson has attributed his ever-changing, multicolored skin to *vitiligo.*

Vitiligo, which is itself believed to be an autoimmune disorder, can also signal other autoimmune diseases besides Graves' disease including diabetes, *pernicious anemia* (a severe form of anemia), *alopecia areata* (see Chapter 1), and *Addison's disease,* a condition in which the adrenal glands malfunction. (See **Dark Patches,** below, and Appendix I.)

Black-and-Blue Marks

Anyone who's ever bumped a leg or arm on a sharp corner knows what a bruise—black-and-blue mark—looks like. Medically known as a *contu-*

sion or *ecchymosis,* this distinctive mark is usually benign. It's normally the result of capillaries (tiny blood vessels) breaking, most often from an injury, and blood leaking into the surrounding tissue. If you press one of these bruises with your finger, they don't blanch. Occasionally, leaking blood forms a large clot under the skin, medically known as a *hematoma.*
Besides looking black and blue, the skin may also feel lumpy.

The tendency to bruise easily can be an inherited trait. It's also an annoying but natural sign of growing older; as we age, our skin's protective fat layer thins, allowing the blood vessels to break more easily.

SPEAKING OF SIGNS

The Earth has a skin and that skin has diseases, one of its diseases is called man.

—Friedrich Nietzsche, 19th-century German philosopher

Bruises that are *not* the result of physical trauma are medically known as *purpura.* Like hematomas and other bruises, they're signs that blood is leaking into the tissues under the skin, and they, too, fail to blanch when pressed. The leakage can be a reaction to certain medications, especially blood thinners, such as aspirin and warfarin (Coumadin), and corticosteroids. Some herbal or other dietary supplements, such as ginkgo, ginger, fish oil, and garlic, can also increase the chances of getting black-and-blue marks. These bruises can also signal nutritional deficiencies, such as a lack of vitamin C, K, or B_{12}, folic acid, or bioflavonoids (a compound found most commonly in citrus and other fruits as well as some vegetables).

Frequent or unexplained bruising can be a warning sign of some serious systemic conditions, especially *leukemia.* Other skin signs of leukemia include paleness (see **Pale Skin,** above), fatigue, shortness of breath during physical activity, frequent infections, and unexplained bleeding.

SIGN OF THE TIMES

The Dead Sea has been a haven for skin disease sufferers for centuries. Today, the area is home to dozens of medical facilities specializing in *climatotherapy*—climate therapy—for skin and other diseases. The salty seawater and filtered sunlight are thought to be therapeutic for the skin.

Bruising can signal *Cushing's syndrome* (aka *hypercortisolism*), a disorder in which the adrenal glands produce too much of the hormone cortisol. People with Cushing's usually suffer from weak muscles, severe fatigue, and infertility. Women with this condition often have *hirsutism*—excess hair on their faces, chests, and other places women normally don't have a lot of hair. (See Chapter 1.) They also are frequently obese and have irregular periods.

Very easy and extensive bruising may also be the earliest warning sign of a low blood platelet count—medically known as *thrombocytopenia*—which can be due to several serious conditions such as leukemia and HIV/AIDS. (Platelets, which are produced in the bone marrow, are needed for blood to clot.)

Lots of black-and-blue marks sometimes signal cirrhosis and other liver diseases, *lymphoma* (cancer of the lymphatic system), lupus (see **Butterfly Mask,** above), and hypothyroidism (see Appendix I).

WARNING SIGN

 Numerous black-and-blue marks in various stages of fading may be signs of repeated blows to the skin. This can be an important sign of physical abuse.

Finally, bruising is a common sign of *Ehlers-Danlos syndrome (EDS),* a rare connective tissue disorder primarily affecting the skin, blood vessels, and joints. (See Chapter 7.) The other classic skin sign of EDS is very stretchable skin. Many people with this condition, however, may not have, or may ignore, this or some of its other body signs, which may include hyperflexible joints (see Chapter 7), joint dislocation, scoliosis, and eye problems. Unfortunately, because the signs are often missed or misdiagnosed, an estimated 90% of people with EDS—which is potentially debilitating and life-threatening—go undiagnosed until they seek attention for a medical emergency.

STOP SIGN

 To hasten the healing of a bruise, ice it for 15 minutes each hour for the first day or so. If possible, keep the bruised area raised above the level of the heart.

Purplish Patterns

If your skin has a fishnet, lacy, or crosshatched purplish pattern, you may have the classic sign of the skin condition *livedo reticularis*. This mottled (reticulated) pattern is usually seen on the torso or extremities and is the result of constricting blood vessels. Livedo reticularis often shows up when you go out in the cold, but it doesn't disappear right away when you warm up.

When the lines of the purple pattern are contiguous, like an intact fishnet, it's usually a benign sign. But if many of the lines are disconnected, it can be an early warning sign of a number of systemic diseases, including rheumatoid arthritis, rheumatic fever, lupus, and *thrombocythemia*. This last is a condition in which there are too many blood platelets; it shouldn't be confused with thrombocytopenia (see **Black-and-Blue Marks**, above), a condition in which there are too few platelets.

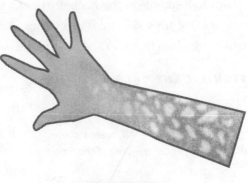

MOTTLED SKIN
(Livedo Reticularis)

Livedo reticularis is often the first sign of *antiphospholipid antibody syndrome (APS)* (see **Dark Stripes**, above), a coagulation disorder that can cause a blood clot *(thrombosis)* in the arteries or veins. These clots raise the risk of seizures, strokes, heart attacks, and pulmonary emboli.

Also known as *Hughes' syndrome*, APS is also a risk factor for recurrent miscarriages. In fact, it's responsible for about 20% of recurrent miscarriages.

WARNING SIGN

People with livedo, whether or not they have APS, are at increased risk of recurrent miscarriages. If you have these purple skin patterns and are pregnant or have had a history of miscarriage, mention it to your doctor.

Dark Patches

If you have dark patches on your body rather than your face and they're thicker or more velvety than normal skin, it may signal a type of hyperpigmentation medically known as *acanthosis nigricans (AN)*. When they first notice it, people with AN often complain that they have a dirty area on their skin that doesn't seem to wash off. The patches range in color from tan to dark brown and in size from very small to quite large. They're most often found on the back of the neck, the armpits, the groin, or in any of the body's skin folds or creases. Another sign of AN is *skin tags,* which are often found in and around the patches. (See **Skin Tags,** below.)

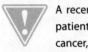

SIGNIFICANT FACT

A recent study found that in patients with both AN and cancer, the AN preceded the diagnosis of cancer one-third of the time.

AN is sometimes inherited and is most common among those of African decent. These skin discolorations usually develop slowly.

AN can be a reaction to certain drugs, including corticosteroids, oral contraceptives, human growth hormone, and insulin. More commonly, it's seen in people who are obese, in which case it may point to insulin resistance. It's often an important early warning sign of diabetes. In overweight women, it can be a tip-off to *polycystic ovarian syndrome* (*PCOS*), the most common hormonal disorder in women of reproductive age and a leading cause of infertility. (See Chapter 1.) AN is also sometimes seen in people with Cushing's syndrome, a hormone disorder of the adrenal glands. (See **Black-and-Blue Marks,** above).

Dark patches on the skin, especially on the knuckles, nipples, underarms, pubic area, and in skin creases, can also signal other disorders of the adrenal glands, such as *Addison's disease,* a condition in which the adrenal glands fail to function properly. (See **Large White Patches,** above, and Appendix I.)

Unlike the localized patches of AN, the dark patches of Addison's tend to be scattered around the body. They usually show up on sun-exposed areas but may also be found under the arms, around the nipples, on the palms and soles, around the genitals and anus, and even in the mouth. If you have dark patches in your mouth as well as on your skin, it's a pretty sure sign you have Addison's. Other signs of Addison's include vitiligo (see **Large White Patches,** above), pubic and underarm hair loss in women, weakness, weight loss, and gastrointestinal problems. Unfortunately, Addison's is a very underdiagnosed condition; without treatment, it can be life-threatening.

AN can also be an early warning sign of stomach or other gastrointestinal cancers. People with cancer-related AN tend to be thinner and older than those with noncancerous AN, and their dark patches usually develop very quickly.

Reddish Patches

Having multiple red patches on your skin may be a passing benign skin problem such as pimples or prickly heat. Or it can signal a more problematic, persistent condition. For example, a crop of raised red patches with silvery scales can be a sign of *psoriasis*. The psoriasis patches are often found spread over the scalp, elbows, knees, back, and buttocks.

Psoriasis is thought to be an autoimmune disease and tends to run in families. While this condition can last a lifetime, some psoriasis suffers have long periods without flare-ups. About 20% of people with this chronic skin disease also have arthritis—medically known as *psoriatic arthritis*. In some people psoriasis is an early warning sign of arthritis, while in others the joint problems come first.

SIGNIFICANT FACT

The fact that fair-skinned people get sunburned easily isn't the only reason they're at increased risk for skin cancer. Another contributing factor is that they tend not to tan. Skin turns tan because of an increase in melanin, which protects the skin from dangerous rays. Scientists are now experimenting with drugs that, when applied to the skin, can safely increase melanin and produce a tan indoors, which will protect the skin outdoors.

On the other hand, a single reddish, rough, or scaly patch may be a warning sign of *solar keratosis* (aka *actinic keratosis*), a precancerous condition. (It's possible to have more than one of these precancerous spots.) The patch or patches can also be dark pink or even skin-colored, in which case you're more likely to feel than see them. If not removed, solar keratosis can turn into *squamous cell carcinoma (SCC)*.

SCC is the second most common type of skin cancer. *Basal cell carcinoma (BCC)* is the most common, and *melanoma* is the rarest but most deadly. (See **Lumps and Bumps**, below.) SCCs are usually red, inflamed, and crusty or scaly patches that have irregular borders. They may be slightly raised and wart-like, break open (*ulcerate*), bleed, and often fail to heal.

Like all skin cancers, SCC is due mainly to exposure to ultraviolet (UV) rays from the sun or from tanning parlors. The carcinogenic effects of UV rays from any source are cumulative.

Skin cancers are most often seen on the face, neck, bald scalp, hands, shoulders, arms, and back—all places that are often exposed to the sun. The chest area exposed by V-neck shirt is a common site for skin cancer. The rim of the ear and the lower lip are vulnerable to these cancers as well. As with other skin cancers, people with light skin, hair, and eyes have the greatest risk. Those who freckle easily but tend not to tan are at increased risk. Dark-skinned people, especially those of African descent, are less likely to get skin cancer than whites. But when they do get skin cancer, it's more likely to be SCC than either BCC or melanoma.

Regardless of skin tone, SCC can occur on skin that's been injured from burns, scars, sores that don't readily heal, and sites previously exposed to a large number of X-rays or certain toxic chemicals. In addition,

SIGN OF THE TIMES

Jane Austen and President John F. Kennedy suffered from Addison's disease. Kennedy never admitted to the public that he had this potentially fatal illness. At age 27, singer Helen Reddy was also diagnosed with Addison's. She's become a patron of the Australian Addison's Disease Association.

SIGNIFICANT FACT

Skin cancer is the only cancer that's almost totally preventable. Yet 1 in 6 people in the United States will develop skin cancer.

conditions that cause chronic skin inflammation or suppress the immune system over an extended period put a person at risk for SCC.

WARNING SIGN

 Recent studies have found that excessive alcohol consumption appears to increase the risk of developing melanoma, especially in women.

Although slow-growing, if not treated the patch can invade surrounding tissue, resulting in serious damage and disfigurement. And it can spread into the lymph nodes and other parts of the body, where it can be life-threatening.

WARNING SIGN

 SCCs that first arise on the ear, on the lower lip, or in the mouth are the ones most likely to spread.

SCC, as well as an early form of this skin cancer known as *Bowen's disease* (aka *squamous cell carcinoma in situ*), can also be reactions to immunosuppressive therapy, particularly following organ transplantation and treatment of diabetes and other chronic illnesses.

Bowen's disease can also signal the presence of *human papillomavirus (HPV)*, especially when it appears on the genitals. The classic sign of Bowen's disease is sore or weathered-looking skin. Compared with those of actinic keratosis, Bowen's disease patches tend to be crusty and larger (often over a half inch), redder, and scalier.

STOP SIGN

 To help prevent skin cancer:
- Avoid direct exposure to the sun between 10:00 A.M. and 4:00 P.M.
- Avoid sun lamps and tanning beds.
- Be sure to reapply sunscreen every 2 hours.
- Wear long sleeves, a hat, and sunglasses when out in the sun.
- Apply SPF 15 or higher, broad-spectrum sunscreen, which protects against both UVA and UVB.

Red Palms

If you notice the palms of your hands are always red but not sore, you may have a *palmar erythema.* This may be a totally benign condition, or it can signal a vitamin B deficiency or heavy alcohol consumption. Indeed, red palms can be red flags for alcohol-related cirrhosis of the liver, as well as hepatitis and other liver diseases. They can also signal hyperthyroidism, diabetes, rheumatoid arthritis, tuberculosis, and even cancer.

Painless, flat, red spots on the palms of your hands may be a very rare condition called *Janeway lesions.* (They also appear on the soles of the feet.) Janeway lesions are telltale signs of *infective endocarditis,* an inflammation of the lining of the heart, which can lead to heart failure, blood clots, and stroke. The infection can come from anything from IV drug use to dental or heart surgery. Other skin signs of endocarditis are red, painful nodules on the fingers and toes—medically known as *Osler's nodes*—and hemorrhages under the nails (see **Dark Stripes,** above) and on the whites of the eyes *(Roth spots).* Edema and excessive sweating are signs that the infection is worsening.

Scaly Rash on Palms or Soles

If you notice a lot of little scales on the palms of your hands or soles of your feet, you may mistake them for a cluster of warts or even psoriasis. (See **Reddish Patches,** above.) But you may have *Reiter's syndrome* (aka *reactive arthritis*), an inflammation of the joints that mostly affects young adult men. (See **Pitted Nails,** above.) The lesions—medically known as *keratosis blennorrhagica*—may look reddish or yellow-brown and occasionally clump into crusty plaques that have peeling edges. Other signs of Reiter's syndrome—which can result from some sexually transmitted diseases or from intestinal infections—include eye infections and painful urination.

These lesions may also signal *postular psoriasis* of the palms and

SIGNIFICANT FACT

Approximately 30 to 50% of people with diabetes develop some form of skin disease.

soles, a rare form of psoriasis, which can be a reaction to certain medications or chemicals such as steroids, lithium, penicillin, and iodine. This condition can also be triggered by infections and emotional stress.

SPOTS AND VEINS

Small Red Raised Spots

If you start noticing small red or violet, slightly raised, smooth, rounded spots popping up on your torso, you may have *Campbell de Morgan* spots (aka *cherry angiomas*). The spots may look like red domes and are usually smaller than $\frac{1}{4}$ inch.

Campbell de Morgan spots are a common benign sign of aging that tend to occur in men and women in their 40s and 50s. Because they often increase with age, they used to be called *senile angiomas*. The spots are actually overgrowths of blood vessels in the skin. When pressed, they don't blanch. They're usually totally harmless, but may be of cosmetic concern to some.

Freckles and Other Tiny Spots

Most of us assume that if we see small dark spots on someone's skin, they're freckles. Medically known as *ephelides,* freckles are deposits of excess skin pigment (*melanin*) on the skin and can be red, brown, tan, or black. They're usually benign, sometimes inherited, and most often seen in fair-skinned people when they're exposed to the sun. As the sun fades in the winter, the freckles are likely to follow. But sometimes a freckle is more than meets the eye.

For example, if you spot very dark or black freckle-like spots that don't fade, it can be a telltale sign of

SIGN OF THE TIMES

Fashionable ancient Roman women and men applied faux "beauty marks" on their faces, necks, shoulders, and arms. Beauty marks were also very popular in the 17th and 18th centuries and were often fashioned out of fancy fabrics such as taffeta and Spanish leather. The placement of the patches was often used to indicate one's political leaning.

Addison's disease (see **Dark Patches,** above, and Appendix I). These tiny spots are usually found on the face (especially the forehead) and the shoulders.

On the other hand, if you have pinpoint red, purple, or brown spots *under* the skin—that is, subcutaneously—they're not freckles at all.

Rather, these are *petechiae,* or tiny hemorrhages. These subcutaneous dots usually start out red and then turn purplish or brown before fading.

Petechiae are a type of telangiectasia, those tiny dilated blood vessels visible under the skin. (See **Rosy Cheeks,** above.) Like purpura (see **Black-and-Blue Marks,** above)—which are actually large clumps of petechiae—they don't blanch or disappear when pressed. These tiny spots commonly occur on the face, legs, arms, and even in the mouth. They can, however, occur anywhere on the body, including on the genitals.

Both petechiae and purpura can signal a low blood platelet count. They may be a reaction to certain medications such the blood thinners aspirin and Coumadin, and corticosteroids, which can interfere with platelet production. They can also be a revealing sign of an autoimmune disorder or diseases that affect bone marrow, such as leukemia, HIV/AIDS, certain forms of anemia, and some viral infections.

Petechiae and purpura are classic signs of *idiopathic thrombocytopenic purpura (ITP),* an autoimmune bleeding disorder also characterized by low levels of platelets. (See **Black-and-Blue Marks,** above.) In addition to skin spots, other ITP signs include easy bruising, prolonged bleeding from cuts, spontaneous bleeding from the nose or gums, blood in the urine or stools, and heavy periods.

IPT is 2 to 3 times more likely to strike women than men, and it's more likely to affect younger women (between the ages of 12 and 25) than older ones. In fact, many women with ITP suffer from heavy menstrual bleeding. Fortunately, this condition rarely causes cerebral hemorrhages. But when it does, it can be life-threatening.

Spider Spots

Seeing a spider on your skin can certainly be terrifying, but spotting a spidery-looking mark can give you a creepy-crawly feeling as well. Medically known as *spider nevi* (aka *spider angioma, vascular spider,* and *nevus araneus*), these are small, abnormal clusters of blood vessels just below the skin surface. They usually have a red spot in the center that looks like a spider's head and spidery extensions radiating outward. These spider spots are the most common form of telangiectasia and are usually found on the face and upper body. They shouldn't be confused with *spider veins,* which are small varicose veins commonly found on the legs. (See **Small Leg Veins**, below.)

Unlike petechiae and Campbell de Morgan spots (see **Small Red Raised Spots**, above), which do not blanch when pressed, spider nevi momentarily turn white or disappear when pressure is applied to them.

Spider nevi are often benign and can be a sign of early pregnancy. However, they can signal some systemic conditions, including cirrhosis of the liver and other liver diseases, rheumatoid arthritis, and hyperthyroidism. (See Appendix I.)

VISIBLE VEINS

Small Leg Veins

If you notice small, raised blood vessels near the surface of the skin on your legs, it's most likely *spider veins,* which are smaller versions of varicose veins. (See **Large Leg Veins**, below.) Spider veins are usually found on the thighs, calves, and ankles. They may look like a sunburst, a spider-web, or a tree branch.

Spider veins sometimes run in families and are more common in women than men. Usually benign, they can pop up during puberty, pregnancy, or when on birth control pills or hormone replacement therapy. Being overweight is another risk factor, as is wearing hosiery that cuts off the circulation.

Large Leg Veins

While spider veins are small, red, or purplish, *varicose veins* are large, raised, twisted, and blue, and the area around them may itch or ache. They can be inherited, or a sign of pregnancy, obesity, or hormonal changes. Or they can simply be a warning sign that you've been on

SPEAKING OF SIGNS

Varicose veins are the result of an improper selection of grandparents.
—William Osler, the Father of Modern Medicine

your feet too long. As with spider veins, they can also be a telltale sign that you're wearing socks or stockings that are too tight. It's not unusual for a person to have both spider veins and varicose veins.

Although usually just a cosmetic concern, varicose veins can put you at increased risk for a type of skin ulcer called *venous stasis ulcers*, which occur when the varicose vein prevents the skin from receiving adequate oxygen. People with varicose veins are also at increased risk for *phlebitis* (aka *thrombophlebitis*), a swelling or inflammation of the veins. Phlebitis usually affects veins in the leg and is caused by blood clots. (See **Purplish Patterns**, above.) Not all veins afflicted by phlebitis are visible. But if you can see the affected vein, it's called *superficial thrombophlebitis*. While this is largely a benign condition, it can cause discomfort. Occasionally, it can be a sign of an abdominal cancer or *deep vein thrombosis (DVT)*. (See Chapter 7.)

In DVT, a clot forms in a vein located deep within the leg, causing redness, swelling, and pain. If the clot breaks off, it can lodge in the lungs, causing a life-threatening *pulmonary embolism;* sometimes the clot will travel to the heart or brain, leading to a heart attack or stroke.

LUMPS AND BUMPS

Most of us have various-sized lumps and bumps on our skin. Like many other skin signs, most are totally benign. But some may signal underlying systemic disorders and diseases, and some may even be cancerous.

Unfortunately, it's not always easy to spot cancerous growths or to distinguish them from benign ones. Skin cancer comes in many shapes, sizes, textures, and colors. Some are flat, some are raised; some ooze, some don't. And they can appear on any part of the body, including the scalp, the soles of the feet, inside the mouth, and even around or inside the rectum or vagina.

SIGNIFICANT FACT

 Skin cancer is the number 1 cancer in men over age 50. That's more cases of cancer in men than prostate, lung, and colon cancer combined. And men are twice as likely to develop basal cell carcinoma and three times more likely to develop squamous cell carcinoma than women.

WARNING SIGN

 If you drive with your arm out the window you can be putting yourself at increased risk of skin cancer, researchers at St. Louis University have discovered. They found an increase in skin cancer on the left arm and hand of male drivers.

But some general principles do apply: any lump or bump on the skin (medically known as a *papule*) that changes in size or appearance, bleeds, or doesn't go away may be a sign of skin cancer and should be checked.

WARNING SIGN

 One in three Americans will develop a skin cancer at some time in their lives. Ideally, every adult should have his or her skin examined for skin cancer once a year. The frequency depends on your risk factors, including family history, skin color, age, race, and sun exposure.

For example, if you have a small, shiny, raised papule that slowly enlarges and occasionally bleeds, it may signal *basal cell carcinoma (BCC)*.

Usually BCC growths are painless and their borders are irregular and may be thick and pearly white. To confuse matters, BCCs vary greatly in size and appearance. They can be pink, red, purple, tan, brown, or black. Some are flat patches resembling scars, and some may break open and form scabs. Some grow so slowly it's barely noticeable.

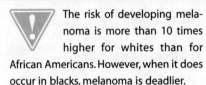

SIGNIFICANT FACT

The risk of developing melanoma is more than 10 times higher for whites than for African Americans. However, when it does occur in blacks, melanoma is deadlier.

BCC is not only the most common form of skin cancer, it's the most common cancer in the United States. The good news is that BCC, which occurs in the outer layer of the skin (*epidermis*), rarely metastasizes. The bad news is that if left untreated, it can invade surrounding tissue, causing serious damage and disfigurement, as well as spread to other organs.

WARNING SIGN

Even if treated successfully, about 25% of people with BCC will have a recurrence within 5 years.

Although they can occur anywhere on the body, BCCs usually develop on the skin that is exposed to the sun, in particular on the face, head, and neck. Being exposed to X-rays and arsenic can also increase the risk.

Multicolored Moles

Many of us have moles, those dark spots that seem to crop up almost anywhere on our bodies. In fact, the average person has between 10 and 40 moles. But if you have lots of moles—100 or more—you are at increased risk of *melanoma*, the least common but most lethal of the skin cancers.

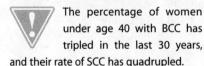

SIGNIFICANT FACT

The percentage of women under age 40 with BCC has tripled in the last 30 years, and their rate of SCC has quadrupled.

Melanomas are usually dark

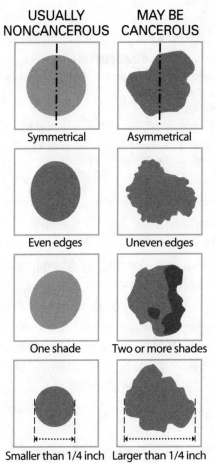

USUALLY NONCANCEROUS | MAY BE CANCEROUS

Symmetrical | Asymmetrical

Even edges | Uneven edges

One shade | Two or more shades

Smaller than 1/4 inch | Larger than 1/4 inch

DETECTING SKIN CANCER

because they grow from pigment-producing skin cells. Although they usually arise from or near a mole or other dark spot, they can sometimes be found on unblemished skin as well. The most common signs of melanoma are a flat, raised, multicolored irregularly shaped mole, either one that is new or one that recently changed appearance.

SIGNIFICANT FACT

Melanoma is on the rise, increasing more rapidly than any other cancer. Its incidence doubled in whites between 1973 and 1995.

Be on the lookout for the **ABCDE**s of melanoma:

A: Asymmetry—one side doesn't look like the other

B: Border is irregular

C: Multicolored

D: Diameter usually larger than the size of a pencil eraser

E: Evolving—can change in size, shape, color and thickness, and can bleed, itch, or crust over

Like other skin cancers, melanomas can take on many different shapes, sizes, colors, and textures. For example, a large brownish spot with darker speckles; an irregular growth with red, white, blue, or blue-black spots; and shiny, firm, dome-shaped bumps can all be melanomas. Although they most often occur on the upper back or face, they can appear anywhere including the limbs, palms, soles, fingertips, and toes, as well as the mucous membranes lining your mouth, nose, vagina, and anus.

Sun exposure is the leading cause of melanoma. Anyone who had blistering sunburns in childhood is at increased risk. In fact, having just one blistering sunburn in childhood doubles the risk of melanoma. And people who use tanning beds or tanning lamps, particularly before age 35, are at increased risk, too.

The good news is that melanoma is highly curable if caught early. If not found in its early stage, however, it can kill quickly.

According to a recent study, the survival rate for foot and ankle melanoma is significantly lower than for leg melanoma.

Waxy, Wart-Like Growths

If you see what looks like brown candle wax on your skin but you haven't been dining by candlelight, it may be a sign of *seborrheic keratosis*. Sometimes referred to as "barnacles" because they look like the barnacles found stuck on logs and seashells, these growths are often mistaken for warts. Indeed, some people call them *seborrheic warts*. But they're not warts: they don't contain HPV, the virus responsible for warts.

Seborrheic keratoses are usually brown but can be black or even flesh-colored. They can be round or oval and as small as ¼ inch up to several inches in width. These growths usually show up on sun-exposed areas—the face, shoulders, back, and chest. Some people have only a single growth, but some have many scattered over their bodies. The edges of these growths are usually not attached to the skin, and they can easily be picked off. Because they tend to itch, people may scratch them off, thus risking an infection.

SIGNIFICANT FACT

Most melanomas are self-discovered or found by family or friends rather than by physicians. But of the patients with doctor-detected melanomas, those whose cancers were diagnosed by dermatologists rather than by other doctors had higher survival rates.

As we age, we tend to get more of these annoying and unsightly growths. In fact, they're the most common benign tumor found in older people. These lesions are sometimes mistaken for skin cancer, especially melanoma. The good news is that they're not cancerous. The bad news is that SCC and melanoma (see **Lumps and Bumps** and **Multicolored Moles,** above) sometimes grow inside them.

Skin Tags

If you notice some small, ugly, movable, skin-colored growths that look like they're hanging on a tiny thread, you have *skin tags*—medically known as *acrochordons*. They often peek out from under skin folds, such as around the neck, under the armpits, in the groin, and under the breasts. But they can crop up on other spots of your body as well.

SIGNIFICANT FACT

Melanoma is one of the more common cancers found in younger people. In fact, 1 in 30,000 girls and 1 in 15,000 boys between the ages of 15 and 19 will develop melanoma.

Many of us are tagged with these telltale, unsightly signs of weight gain and aging. They usually start sprouting when we're in our 30s, and most people have them by the time they reach their 70s.

Overweight people and pregnant women seem to get them more often than others.

Although these growths can be cosmetically compromising, they're not cancerous. Sometimes skin tags will bleed and even become infected if you cut or rip them off.

It used to be believed that skin tags were signs of colon polyps. But there's new evidence that they're more likely to be signs of non-insulin-dependent diabetes and obesity.

Small Yellow Bumps

A bump just under the surface of the skin that is soft and yellow, with a distinct border, is most likely a fat deposit medically known as a *xanthoma*. Xanthomas can range from very small to more than 3 inches in diameter. These fat deposits can signal elevated blood lipid levels, particularly inherited kinds, as well as heart disease, diabetes, primary biliary cirrhosis, and some types of cancer.

SIGN OF THE TIMES

In Italy, legend has it that the navel of Venus, goddess of love, is the model for the popular pasta tortellini.

If found on the eyelids, the most common site for these fat deposits, they are medically called *xanthelasmas*. (See Chapter 2.) Other possible sites for xanthomas are the elbows, joints, tendons, hands, feet, or buttocks. Both xanthelasmas and xanthomas are usually benign. But they can signal high cholesterol levels, a serious risk factor for heart disease.

Movable Lumps

Feeling round, very movable, rubbery lumps under your skin, particularly on the neck, trunk, and forearms, can be disconcerting. But these are likely to be *lipomas,* which are harmless (unless they begin to impinge on a nerve), noncancerous fatty tumors. In fact, lipomas are the most common benign soft-tissue tumor in adults. (See Chapter 6.) They're usually slow-growing and usually don't get any bigger than 2 or 3 inches in diameter. Some people develop only a single growth; some may have multiple lipomas. The people who get them most are women and those who are overweight.

A painless, soft, movable, slow-growing lump could also be a *sebaceous cyst*. (See Chapter 6.) Although these cysts are often found around the neck, they can pop up almost anywhere on the body, including the skin of the scrotum and vagina. Unlike lipomas, these bumps usually have a blackhead-like spot in the middle. They're totally benign, though sometimes they can pop open and ooze.

Belly Button Bump

If you've ever contemplated your navel, you've probably noticed whether it's an "innie" or an "outie." Although both types are perfectly normal, about 90% of navels are "innies." The belly button—which is medically known as the *umbilicus*—is actually a birth scar; when a baby's umbilical cord falls off, a permanent scar forms.

A previously "innie" belly button that has recently become an "outie" is a common sign of pregnancy, especially during the 2nd trimester. If you're not pregnant or are a man, a newly bulging belly button can signal an *umbilical hernia,* a condition in which part of the intestine protrudes through a hole or weakness in the abdominal wall. (When it occurs in the groin area, it's called an *inguinal hernia.*)

Umbilical hernias are very common in infancy but can occur during adulthood, often as a result of obesity, multiple pregnancies, heavy lifting, or even coughing. When the hernia can be pushed back in place by a doctor, it's usually a benign sign. However, a hernia can also become *strangulated* or *incarcerated,* both very painful and potentially life-threatening situations.

If you notice a belly button bump that's inside the navel, irregularly shaped, and possibly with visible blood vessels, it may a sign of *Sister Joseph's nodule* (aka *Sister Mary Joseph's nodule*). This rare lump is usually painless and firm but may ooze. It can be bluish violet, brownish red, or even white.

Unfortunately, Sister Joseph's nodule usually signifies an advanced cancer in the abdominal cavity, but the malignancy can occur in virtually any organ. In some cases, the Sister Joseph's nodule is the only sign of an ovarian, colorectal, or pancreatic cancer.

SIGN OF THE TIMES

In 1912 Sister Mary Joseph, a surgical assistant to Dr. William Mayo, founder of the Mayo Clinic, identified the nodule that now bears her name. Ten years before the nodule was named for her, Sister Joseph, as she became known, died at age 82 of bronchopneumonia. According to several sources, she noticed a nodule on her own navel shortly before her death.

TEXTURE CHANGES

Stripes on the Skin

For some of us, the handwriting might be on the wall. But for others, the handwriting's actually on their skin—they can write words on their skin by lightly scratching it with their nails or a sharp pointed object. Medically known as *dermographism* (or *dermatographism*), which literally means "writing on the skin," this condition is in fact the most common form of a type of hives called *physical urticaria*. It's caused by histamine—the same substance that causes the sneezing and running nose of allergies—being released by pressure on the skin. The histamine can cause swelling, redness, and itching. In response to a mere scratch, a linear welt or wheal will trace the path of the scratch. The welt can last from half an hour to as long as three hours, and it may itch. Although anyone can get dermographism, it's most common among young adults. It may be a sign of stress, a thyroid condition, or a previous viral infection.

If the lines on your skin are parallel, pink, purplish, or white and don't come and go, you have stretch marks—medically termed *striae*. They're usually found on the abdomen, buttocks, breasts, thighs, and arms. As their name implies, they're signs of rapid or persistent skin stretching. This can happen to adolescents when they have growth spurts, or anyone else when they grow fat. Stretch marks are both hallmarks and permanent records of pregnancy. In fact, 90% of pregnant women have them.

Stretch marks are also frequently found on the shoulders of bodybuilders. Stretch marks on the face, as well as the rest of the body, can signal long-term use or abuse of oral or topical corticosteroids. They can also be signs of such systemic conditions as diabetes, Ehlers-Danlos syndrome (EDS), and Cushing's syndrome. (See **Black-and-Blue Marks,** above.)

WARNING SIGN

According to a recent study, women with stretch marks—whether or not they've been pregnant or obese—are at increased risk for pelvic prolapse in later life. In pelvic prolapse, the structures that support the organs of the pelvis weaken, causing pressure, pain, and urinary and/or rectal incontinence. Sometimes a woman can actually see or feel a bulge in her vagina.

Thick, Hard Skin

If your skin feels hard and taut, it may be a sign of a serious autoimmune disorder, *scleroderma,* which means "hard skin" in Latin. Caused by an overproduction of collagen, scleroderma is a chronic connective tissue disorder that can cause the skin of the face, hands, and fingers to thicken and harden. Unfortunately, the joints and internal organs can also be affected. Scleroderma often goes hand in hand with *Raynaud's disease,* a condition that causes the hands and fingers to turn blue. (See Chapter 7.)

Scleroderma, also known as *systemic sclerosis,* occurs in women 4 times more often than in men. In its mildest form—called *limited scleroderma*—facial and finger skin becomes shiny and uncomfortably tight. Telangiectasia (tiny, dilated blood vessels) is another common skin sign of limited scleroderma.

SIGNIFICANT FACT

CREST is the acronym for the signs of *limited scleroderma*

C: Calcium deposits under the skin and in the body

R: Raynaud's disease

E: Esophageal dysfunction

S: Skin damage on the fingers or toes *(sclerodactyly)*

T: *Telangiectasia* (dilated blood vessels)

The more serious form—called *diffuse scleroderma*—affects the major internal organs. It can cause gastrointestinal or swallowing problems and can be life threatening.

Red or Purple Hard Patches

If you find thick or hard, sometimes oval, red or purple patches on your skin, they may be signs of *morphea,* a rare autoimmune skin condition typically found on the torso and extremities. These patches may gradually turn yellow and develop a whitish spot in the center. They may be slightly depressed and look like an unhealed burn or wound. Morphea (the word means "form" or "structure" in Greek) is seen more often in women than men.

Morphea is actually a localized form of *scleroderma,* an autoimmune disease that can cause serious internal organ damage. (See **Thick, Hard Skin,** above.) The good news is that morphea affects only the skin and not the internal organs. As in scleroderma, though, the skin can harden, thicken, and become less flexible, resulting in impaired dexterity and mobility.

SIGN OF THE TIMES

The term *cellulite* was first coined in France more than 150 years ago. It made its way across the Atlantic by the 1960s, and has stuck.

Lumpy, Dimply Skin

You may have noticed unattractive soft lumpy dimples on your own or someone else's thighs and buttocks. These soft lumps and bumps are signs of the dreaded cellulite—medically known as *adiposis edematosa* or *dermopanniculosis deformans.* Also sometimes graphically dubbed in the medical literature as the *mattress phenomenon, orange peel syndrome,* and *cottage cheese skin,* cellulite is seen almost exclusively in women. (It shouldn't be confused with *cellulitis,* an inflammation of the connective tissue of the skin.)

SIGNIFICANT FACT

Dimples on the face are fairly common, but if you notice a dimple on your leg, arm, or torso, it may be a sign that your mother had amniocentesis when she was pregnant with you, and you were punctured by the needle. This sign has been seen much less frequently since sonograms have made it easier to guide the needles during amniocentesis.

Cellulite is normal fat tissue beneath the skin; it tends to increase with age. The evidence is slim that weight gain causes cellulite—in fact, up to 98% of all women, including very thin women, have this condition. However, cellulite is more visible on heavy women. And there is some evidence that weight gain can make it worse, as can a sedentary lifestyle and oral contraceptives.

The good news is this unappealing sign is totally benign in women. In men, however, cellulite may be a sign of androgen deficiency from such conditions as Klinefelter's syndrome. (See Chapters 1 and 7.) Men who are on estrogen hormone therapy for prostate cancer sometimes get cellulite.

Wrinkles

Wrinkles are the one skin sign that we all will develop if we live long enough. But wrinkles aren't just signs of aging. While the degree to which we wrinkle is determined genetically to some extent, wrinkles are also revealing signs of our lifestyles.

For example, wrinkles can be a telltale sign that you've spent a lot of time in the sun without skin protection, or that you've been

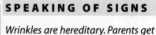

SPEAKING OF SIGNS

Wrinkles are hereditary. Parents get them from their children.

—American actress and singer Doris Day

overexposed to certain toxic chemicals. Wrinkles can also be a dead giveaway that a person is or has been a heavy drinker or smoker. Indeed, smoking, especially in women, can be particularly damaging to the skin because it depletes estrogen, hastening both skin aging and menopause.

If a smoker doesn't already have a lung disease, having very wrinkled skin can be a warning

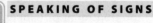

SPEAKING OF SIGNS

Wrinkles should merely indicate where smiles have been.

—Mark Twain, 19th-century American author and humorist

sign that he or she is at increased risk of developing a serious one, especially *emphysema* or other *chronic obstructive pulmonary disease* (*COPD*). (See **Bluish Skin**, above.)

SIGNING OFF

Many diseases and disorders can first be spotted on the skin in the form of nodules, papules, pustules, patches, and petechiae, to name a few. Many of these skin signs may seem at first sight to be simply cosmetically displeasing. But they shouldn't necessarily be ignored or covered over.

Obviously, any skin or nail sign that involves excessive itching, swelling, bleeding, pain, or pus should be checked out by a doctor right away. But when dealing with any skin and nail signs, ruling out a cancer should always be a top priority. The rule of thumb is that *any* change in the size, shape, texture, or color of a mark should be immediately reported to a doctor, preferably a dermatologist. The following doctors may be involved in diagnosing and treating the underlying causes or consequences of skin diseases:

- *Allergist/Immunologist:* A medical doctor who specializes in the diagnosis and treatment of allergies and immune system disorders.
- *Dermatologist:* A medical doctor who has special training in diseases of the skin and nails.
- *Endocrinologist:* A medical doctor who specializes in diagnosing and treating hormone-related diseases and disorders.
- *Hematologist:* A medical doctor who specializes in diagnosing and treating diseases of the blood.
- *Oncologist:* A medical doctor who specializes in the diagnosis and treatment of cancer.
- *Plastic surgeon:* A medical doctor who repairs or reconstructs visible parts of the body.
- *Rheumatologist:* A medical doctor who focuses on inflammatory and degenerative diseases.

BODY SIGNS REVIEW

MULTISYSTEM DISEASES AND THEIR SIGNS

Many potentially serious diseases often affect several different and seemingly unrelated body parts and systems. Because of this, many of these disorders are often under- or misdiagnosed, or at the very least their diagnosis is delayed. And the fact that some of the signs of these conditions are subtle compounds the problem.

The following is a list of some of the more common multisystem diseases and their signs, both the classic ones and those that are more unusual. If you do have one of these conditions, you may have many or only a few of its body signs. Regardless of the number of signs you have, if you're at all concerned, discuss it with your physician.

ADDISON'S DISEASE

Addison's disease (*adrenal insufficiency* or *hypocortisolism*) is a rare disorder in which the adrenal glands produce too little of the stress hormone cortisol, and sometimes other important hormones. This potentially life-threatening disease most commonly strikes adults between the ages of 30 and 50.

Signs of Addison's disease may include:

- Muscle weakness and fatigue
- Craving for salt and salty foods
- Skin color changes in the mouth (*oral mucosal melanosis*)
- Darkening of the skin
- White patches on the skin (*vitiligo*)
- Thinning hair
- Supersensitivity to smell (*hyperosmia*)
- Decreased appetite and weight loss
- Nausea and vomiting
- Irritability and depression
- Slow, sluggish movement

CUSHING'S SYNDROME

Cushing's syndrome (*hypercortisolism*) is a condition in which the adrenal glands produce too much of the stress hormone cortisol. Both women and men can have Cushing's, and it usually strikes between the ages of 20 and 50.

Signs of Cushing's syndrome may include:

- "Moon face" (red, round, and full)
- "Buffalo hump" (fatty deposits between the shoulders)
- Protruding stomach
- Central obesity
- Thin arms and legs
- Muscle weakness and fatigue
- Increased thirst
- Increased urination
- Stretch marks
- Easy bruising
- Dark patches on the skin (*acanthosis nigricans*)
- Excessive facial and body hair in women (*hirsutism*)
- Lack of menstruation (*amenorrhea*)
- Infertility
- Impotence in men
- Decreased sex drive in both sexes

DIABETES

Diabetes is a disease in which the body does not produce or properly use insulin, a hormone that is needed to convert sugar, starches, and other food into energy needed for daily life. It's estimated that more than 20 million Americans have diabetes; unfortunately, more than 6 million of them don't know it. Diabetes is the leading cause of new cases of blindness and of kidney failure in American adults. And having diabetes greatly increases the risk of suffering a heart attack or stroke.

The signs of diabetes may include:

- Excessive hunger
- Excessive thirst
- Frequent urination
- Weight loss
- Fatigue and weakness
- Eye or vision changes
- Hair loss
- Frequent infections
- Slow-healing cuts and bruises
- Tingling or numbness (*paresthesia*) in feet and occasionally hands
- Sweet- or alcohol-smelling breath
- Hair loss
- Gum disease
- Dry mouth
- Discolored tongue
- Taste distortions
- Sweet-smelling urine
- Tea-colored urine
- Profuse sweating, especially at night
- Red palms
- White patches on the skin (*vitiligo*)
- Dark patches on the skin (*acanthosis nigricans*)
- Thick nails or other nail changes

HEART ATTACK

A heart attack (*myocardial infarction*) occurs when the blood supply to part of the heart muscle is interrupted or stopped because one or more of the heart's arteries is blocked. An estimated 1.2 million Americans suffered a heart attack in 2007; more than 450,000 were estimated to have died from it.

The signs of a heart attack may occur suddenly and cause intense discomfort. But some start slowly, can be mild, and may not even be obviously heart-related. They may include:

- Chest pressure, discomfort, or pain
- Discomfort or pain in other areas of the upper body
- Pain or discomfort in one, usually the left, or both arms, the back, neck, jaw, or stomach
- Shortness of breath, which may occur with or without chest discomfort
- Impending sense of doom
- Cold sweat
- Nausea and vomiting
- Light-headedness
- Fainting

HYPERTHYROIDISM

Hyperthyroidism—sometimes called overactive thyroid or *thyrotoxicosis*—is a condition in which the thyroid gland produces too much of the thyroid hormone thyroxine, which is responsible for metabolism. Graves' disease, which affects more women than men, is the most common form of hyperthyroidism.

Hyperthyroidism can produce a wide variety of body signs, including:

- Rapid heart rate
- Increased thirst
- Increased appetite
- Rapid weight loss
- Irritability
- Nervousness and emotional instability
- Insomnia

- Hand tremors
- Heat intolerance
- Excessive sweating
- Staring, bulging eyes
- Eyes that dart back and forth (*nystagmus*)
- Dry eyes
- Muscle weakness
- Goiter (enlarged thyroid gland)
- Hair loss
- Frequent bowel movements
- Menstrual irregularities
- Enlarged breasts in men

HYPOTHYROIDISM

Hypothyroidism—sometimes called underactive thyroid—is a condition in which the thyroid gland produces inadequate amounts of the thyroid hormone thyroxine, the hormone responsible for metabolism. More women than men are likely to be hypothyroid, and it tends to strike after the age of 50.

Signs of hypothyroidism may include:
- Dry, coarse hair
- Thin, brittle nails
- Dry, pale skin
- Hair loss
- Puffy face
- Droopy eyes (*ptosis*)
- Cold intolerance
- Constipation
- Weight gain
- Edema
- Hoarse, slow speech
- Sleepiness
- Fatigue
- Depression
- Irregular or abnormal menstrual periods

LUPUS

Lupus—medically known as *systemic lupus erythematosus (SLE)*—is a chronic, inflammatory autoimmune disorder that may affect the skin, joints, kidneys, and other organs. Lupus, as it's commonly known, may be mild, or it may be severe enough to cause death. Nine out of 10 people with lupus are women. While it may occur at any age, it most often occurs in people between the ages of 10 and 50. African Americans and Asians are affected more often than people of other races.

Signs of lupus may include:
- Joint pain and swelling
- Red ("butterfly") rash across the nose and cheeks
- Rash on the ears, upper arms, shoulders, chest, and hands
- Rash develops or worsens from sun exposure *(photosensitivity)*
- *Petechiae* (tiny, pinpoint dots from broken blood vessels)
- Fever
- Fatigue
- General discomfort
- Digestive problems
- Mouth ulcers
- Shortness of breath *(dyspnea)*
- Chest pain
- Seizures
- Swollen glands
- Muscle aches
- Nausea and vomiting
- Cold hands and feet *(Raynaud's disease)*
- Numbness and tingling *(paresthesia)*

MYASTHENIA GRAVIS

Myasthenia gravis is an autoimmune neuromuscular disease. It's characterized by variable weakness of the skeletal (voluntary) muscles of the body, which increases during periods of activity and improves with rest. Although myasthenia gravis occurs in all ethnic groups and in both genders, it most commonly affects young adult women (under 40) and older men (over 60).

Signs of myasthenia gravis may include:

- Droopy eyelids (*ptosis*)
- Weak muscles in arms and legs
- Difficulty getting up from a chair
- Difficulty talking and chewing
- Difficulty breathing
- Drooping head
- Facial paralysis
- Double vision
- Hoarse voice

OVARIAN CANCER

Ovarian cancer is one of the deadliest forms of cancer that affects women. In fact, it's the fifth-leading cause of cancer deaths among women. Although highly curable if it is found early and confined to the ovary, ovarian cancer is often not diagnosed until it has advanced and even spread to other parts of the body.

The signs of ovarian cancer may include:

- Excess facial or body hair (*hirsutism*)
- Abdominal bloating
- Increased abdominal girth
- Gastrointestinal disturbances
- Difficulty eating or feeling full quickly
- Unexplained weight gain or loss
- Pelvic or abdominal discomfort, heaviness, or pain
- Lower back pain
- Abnormal menstrual cycles
- Unexplained vaginal bleeding
- Urinary urgency or frequency
- Pain during intercourse

POLYCYSTIC OVARY SYNDROME

Polycystic ovary syndrome (PCOS)—also known as polycystic ovary disease (PCOD) and Stein-Leventhal syndrome—is a hormonal disorder in which the ovaries become enlarged. PCOS, which affects between 5 and 10% of women, is the most common hormonal disorder of reproductive-age women and a leading cause of infertility.

The signs of PCOS may include:

- Irregular, scanty, or absent periods
- Infertility
- Excessive facial and body hair *(hirsutism)*
- Male-pattern baldness
- Deepening of the voice
- Decreased breast size
- Excessive acne
- Dark patches on the skin *(acanthosis nigricans)*
- Excessive weight gain

SARCOIDOSIS

Sarcoidosis is an inflammatory disorder that most commonly affects the lungs. It can, however, affect other body organs or parts, including the skin, eyes, ears, nose, lymph nodes, heart, and liver.

Signs of sarcoidosis may include:

- Shortness of breath *(dyspnea)*
- Coughing
- Chest pain
- Fatigue
- Fever
- Weight loss
- Vision and other eye problems
- Red rashes on the face and body
- Red lumps, particularly on the legs *(erythema nodosum)*
- Purple patches on the skin
- Puffy, hard, cracked, or scaly lips
- Hoarse voice
- Stiff or achy joints
- Tingling and numbness *(paresthesia)*
- Pitted or spotted nails
- Scaly patches on the face *(lupus pernio)*

SJÖGREN'S SYNDROME

Sjögren's syndrome is a rare autoimmune disease in which the body attacks its moisture-producing glands. If untreated, Sjögren's can severely damage the eyes and adversely affect the digestive system, female reproductive system, kidneys, lungs, and other organs.

Sjögren's affects approximately 4 million Americans, 9 out of 10 of whom are women. It mostly occurs between the ages of 40 and 50.

Signs of Sjögren's may include:
- Dry eyes
- Dry mouth
- Dry nose
- Vaginal dryness
- Dry skin
- Difficulty swallowing
- Hoarseness
- Joint inflammation
- Fatigue
- Fever

STROKE

A stroke occurs when the blood supply to part of the brain is interrupted suddenly *(ischemic stroke)* or when a blood vessel in the brain bursts *(hemorrhagic stroke)*. More women than men suffer strokes. African Americans are more likely than whites to suffer a stroke, and when they do, they tend to suffer them earlier in life and have more severe consequences than whites. Recognizing the signs of stroke and getting treatment early—usually within the first 3 hours after signs appear—can reduce the risk of severe disability and even death.

The signs of a stroke may include the sudden appearance of:
- Numbness and/or weakness, especially on one side of the body
- Severe headache
- Dizziness
- Loss of balance or difficulty walking
- Paralysis, especially on one side of the face or body
- Slurred speech or difficulty speaking

- Difficulty finding words (*aphasia*)
- Difficulty understanding people
- Mental confusion
- Blindness, blurred vision, or double vision in one or both eyes

TRANSIENT ISCHEMIC ATTACK

A transient ischemic attack (TIA) is caused by a temporary reduction in the flow of blood (*ischemia*) to the brain, usually due to a clot. It's often called a mini-stroke because it's similar to a stroke but usually lasts for only a few moments to 24 hours. Although the signs may totally disappear, not only can they recur, but a TIA is often a forewarning of a full-blown stroke.

The signs of a TIA are the same as for a stroke. (See above.)

BODY OF RESOURCES

RECOMMENDED WEBSITES AND BOOKS

In writing this book, we used many different medical and scientific sources including textbooks, journals, and websites sponsored by the National Institutes of Health and other professional organizations. In addition, we found many other consumer-oriented websites and books extremely helpful. Below is a list you, the reader, might also find useful and interesting.

WEBSITES

American Academy of Allergy, Asthma, and Immunology
www.aaaai.org

American Academy of Dermatology
www.aad.org

American Academy of Family Physicians
www.aafp.org

American Academy of Ophthalmology
www.aao.org

American Academy of Orthopaedic Surgeons
www.aaos.org

American Academy of Otolaryngic Allergy
www.aaoaf.org

American Academy of Otolaryngology—Head and Neck Surgery
www.entnet.org

American Academy of Physical Medicine and Rehabilitation
www.aapmr.org

American Academy of Sleep Medicine
www.aasmnet.org

American Association of Clinical Endocrinologists
www.aace.com

American Cancer Society
www.cancer.org

American College of Allergy, Asthma, and Immunology
www.acaai.org

American College of Cardiology
www.acc.org

American College of Gastroenterology
www.acg.gi.org

American College of Obstetricians and Gynecologists
www.acog.com

American College of Rheumatology
www.rheumatology.org

American Diabetes Association
www.diabetes.org

American Gastroenterological Association
www.gastro.org

American Heart Association
www.americanheart.org

American Lung Association
www.lungusa.org

American Orthopaedic Foot and Ankle Society
www.aofas.org

American Osteopathic College of Dermatology
www.aocd.org

American Physical Therapy Association
www.apta.org

American Podiatric Medical Association
www.apma.org

American Society for Reproductive Medicine
www.asrm.org

American Society of Clinical Oncology
www.asco.org

American Society of Plastic Surgeons
www.plasticsurgery.org

American Stroke Association
www.strokeassociation.org

American Thoracic Society
www.thoracic.org

American Thyroid Association
www.thyroid.org

American Urological Association
www.auanet.org

Arthritis Foundation
www.arthritis.org

Crohn's and Colitis Foundation of America
www.ccfa.org

Cushing's Support and Research Foundation
www.csrf.net

Endocrine Society
www.endo-society.org

Foundation for Sarcoidosis Research
www.stopsarcoidosis.org

HeartHealthyWomen
www.hearthealthywomen.org

The Hormone Foundation
www.hormone.org

Lupus Foundation of America
www.lupus.org

Mayo Clinic
www.mayoclinic.com

Medline Plus
www.nlm.nih.gov/medlineplus

Merck Manual Home Edition Online
www.merck.com/mmhe/index.html

Myasthenia Gravis Foundation of America
www.myasthenia.org

National Adrenal Diseases Foundation
www.nadf.us

National Cancer Institute
www.cancer.gov

National Eye Institute
www.nei.nih.gov

National Graves' Disease Foundation
www.ngdf.org

National Heart, Lung, and Blood Institute
www.nhlbi.nih.gov

National Institute of Neurological Disorders and Stroke
www.ninds.nih.gov

National Institute of Arthritis and Musculoskeletal and Skin Diseases
www.niams.nih.gov

National Institute on Aging
www.nia.nih.gov

National Institute on Deafness and Other Communication Disorders
www.nidcd.nih.gov

National Kidney and Urologic Diseases Information Clearinghouse
www.kidney.niddk.nih.gov

National Medical Association
www.nmanet.org

National Osteoporosis Foundation
www.nof.org

National Ovarian Cancer Coalition
www.ovarian.org

National Parkinson Foundation
www.parkinson.org

National Scoliosis Foundation
www.scoliosis.org

National Sleep Foundation
www.sleepfoundation.org

National Women's Health Information Center
www.womenshealth.gov

NIH Osteoporosis and Related Bone Diseases—National Resource
Center
www.niams.nih.gov/bone

North American Menopause Society
www.menopause.org

Polycystic Ovarian Syndrome Association
www.pcosupport.org

Scleroderma Foundation
www.scleroderma.org

Sjögren's Syndrome Foundation
www.sjogrens.org

U.S. Food and Drug Administration
www.fda.gov

U.S. National Library of Medicine
www.pubmed.gov

BOOKS

Adam's Navel: A Natural and Cultural History of the Human Form
Michael Sims
Penguin, 2004

The Body Has a Head
Dr. Gustav Eckstein
Bantam, 1980

The Body in Parts: Fantasies of Corporeality in Early Modern Europe
Edited by David Hillman and Carla Mazzio
Routledge, 1997

The Face: A Natural History
Daniel McNeill
First Back Bay, 2000

The Nose: A Profile of Sex, Beauty, and Survival
Gabrielle Glaser
Atria Books, 2002

Medicine in Quotations
Edited by Edward Huth and T. Jock Murray
American College of Physicians, 2000

The Oxford Companion to the Body
Edited by Colin Blakemore and Sheila Jennett
Oxford University Press, 2001

On Blonds
Joanna Pitman
Bloomsbury, 2003

Rapunzel's Daughters
Rose Weitz
Farrar, Straus and Giroux, 2004

Ovid: The Erotic Poems
Peter Green (Trans.)
Penguin Books, 1982

MY BODY SIGNS CHECKUP CHECKLIST

As you've learned from reading *Body Signs,* your body can churn out an enormous amount of signs, from the banal to the bizarre. Keeping track of your body signs is one way to keep track of your health and help you determine if you're sick or well. Here's a checklist to take with you to your next medical checkup. It will help you become a better diagnostic detective. It's also important to take a list of all the prescription and over-the-counter medicines, including vitamins, supplements, herbs, and analgesics, you are taking. And don't forget to include the dosages, too.

HAIR	
Body Sign Description	**Date First Noticed**

EYES	
Body Sign Description	**Date First Noticed**

EARS	
Body Sign Description	Date First Noticed

NOSE	
Body Sign Description	Date First Noticed

LIPS AND MOUTH	
Body Sign Description	Date First Noticed

JAW, THROAT, AND NECK	
Body Sign Description	Date First Noticed

TORSO AND EXTREMITIES	
Body Sign Description	Date First Noticed

PRIVATE PARTS AND BODY WASTES	
Body Sign Description	Date First Noticed

SKIN AND NAILS	
Body Sign Description	Date First Noticed

MEDICATIONS AND DOSAGES

INDEX

Page numbers of illustrations appear in italics.

ABOUT THE AUTHORS

JOAN LIEBMANN-SMITH, PH.D., is a medical writer and medical sociologist who specializes in health promotion and disease prevention in women and children. She is a past recipient of the American Medical Association's Medical Reporting Award.

Dr. Liebmann-Smith received her B.A. from New York University and her Ph.D. from the Graduate Center of the City University of New York. She is currently a consultant at the Strang Cancer Prevention Center in their Healthy Children/Healthy Futures program.

Her articles have appeared in many national magazines, including *American Health, Ms., Newsweek, Redbook, Self,* and *Vogue,* as well as on various medical websites. Liebmann-Smith and her co-author, Jacqueline Egan, have written two previous books: *The Unofficial Guide to Overcoming Infertility* (1999) and *The Unofficial Guide to Getting Pregnant* (2005). She is also the author of *In Pursuit of Pregnancy* (1989), and wrote a book on women and substance abuse for the National Center on Addiction and Substance Abuse at Columbia University (*Women Under the Influence,* Johns Hopkins University Press, 2006). She has appeared on such national television shows as *The Oprah Winfrey Show* and *The Today Show*.

Dr. Liebmann-Smith sits on the board of directors of the National Council on Women's Health. She holds memberships in the National Association of Science Writers, the American Medical Writers Association, and the American Sociological Association. She lives in New York City with her husband, Richard, whose book, *The James Boys,* will be published by Random House in 2008. They have a 25-year-old daughter, Rebecca, and a rescue cat, Fazelnut.

JACQUELINE NARDI EGAN is a medical journalist who specializes in developing and writing educational programs with and for physicians, allied health professionals, patients, and consumers. Currently, she is the associate editorial director at QD Healthcare Group and Continuing Education Alliance in Greenwich, Connecticut, and is a former medical editor of *Family Health* magazine. She has a daughter, Elizabeth, and two rescue dogs, Coco and Abby. She divides her time between Darien, Connecticut, and Sag Harbor, New York.